Beside the Mountain

Finding Strength and Courage Through
My Father's Early Onset Alzheimer's Disease

Stefania Silvestri

ISBN: 0985727209
ISBN-13: 978-0985727208

Typesetting in Adobe Garamond Pro by Casey Bayer.

For my father

Acknowledgements

While my father was sick, I realized I wanted to write this book. But it takes more, I learned later, than wanting to do something. It takes support, in many forms, to transform an idea into a draft, and a draft into a book.

I was blessed with the opportunity to be taught by several outstanding teachers during my studies at the University of Missouri, Columbia, The Summer Writers Institute at Washington University and Emerson College. Sam Stowers and Ray Ronci, you were the first professors to really give me the confidence I needed to solidify my desire to write. Howard Hinkel, thank you for introducing me to the different forms of nonfiction writing. In your class, I finally heard the voice of this memoir. John Estes, your commitment to helping me during and after my studies showed me how extraordinary a man you are. Kathleen Finneran, if it weren't for your honesty and talent as a writer and teacher, I would never have been able to begin my MFA. You are a beautiful memoirist and I aspire to follow in your footsteps, however small my own may be. Megan Marshall, thank you for your edits and your invaluable feedback. And Douglas Whynott, where do I begin? You gave me my structure and another storyline to examine. You will always be an important figure in my life, a beloved professor and friend.

Thank you as well to the final editors of this book, David McCormack, and Will Myers. Thank you also to Casey Bayer for your editing assistance and final design of the book. And to my friends who assisted with formatting, Rachel Imbriglio and Mina Yun. And thank you Sophia Lazare, Kate Knapp and Dina Barsky, for believing in its merit.

My friends in my life have been instrumental in helping me keep my sanity. Jessie, thank you for the peace you gave me during our talks over coffee at The Grind. Thank you, Marc, for putting up with me day in and day out. I know why you are everyone's favorite. Susan, thank you for the opportunities you gave me, for introducing me to Kathleen, for the meals and the laughter. Meagan, Struby, Sarah—I could never explain to you fully how much I needed you back then. Each of you has such beauty and infinite wisdom. Andi, thank you for the beautiful cover of this book and for keeping that joyful spirit you had when I first met you. The Rallos—Linda, Nick, Sophia, Nathalie and Nicholas—you all are our family, and the love you shared with us during those times I will never forget. Dan, *my* rock, you are a son to my mother, a brother to my sisters and to me; you are and will always be my dearest friend. From everything that I am, I thank you all.

In the end, *Beside the Mountain* made me examine not just my father's illness, but the unique bond my family shares. My brother-in-law Massimo, I am so grateful to have you in our lives, for the nephew I love so dearly, and for the kindness you have shown us. Flavia and Nicole, I know it wasn't easy having me ask you questions and prodding your memories for the moments you would have rather not relived. Thank you for helping me write this book, for the moments you let me cry with you, and the times you comforted me as I complained about Mom's insistence that I continue. But Mom, thank you for that. Thank you for pushing me. Thank you for the timelines and the details, for the glimpses into the moments I never knew of—but that I've tried to recreate. Your strength flows through each of our spirits. You all have helped me create something I am proud of.

And to my nephew Giovanni, your grandfather watches you like he does the rest of us. Each time you smile, I think of him and I imagine he does so in turn.

Preface

Alzheimer's disease affected my family in a way I never expected. For one, I never even imagined it *could* happen to a man who had yet to reach fifty. But it did and it came and it took from me not just my father, but my strength, my hope. At fourteen, I would never have foreseen the ensuing years that would come to pass nor imagined the woman I would later become.

Today, my younger sister Nicole is nearing the end of her bachelor's degree with honors. She has grown into an independent, courageous and determined woman. My older sister Flavia has an MBA and works fulltime. She is also a loving mother and a dutiful wife herself. Her young son and my beautiful nephew is my father's namesake. My mother has continued moving forward with dignity and still in that warrior way since she first became a caretaker. I see that sadness still weighs heavy on her from the years of losing him, but it's a burden we all bear. And me—I decided to pursue a Master of Fine Arts in creative writing and wrote this book which my mother always said I would. Without her persistence, which I fought against at times, I don't believe I would have ever been able to write it.

My wish was to create something beautiful from the pain of my father's loss. The details comprise a truth found within my family's heartache and suffering—that love never once abandoned us. Life, love, family and place are inextricably linked. Yet, so too, in this memoir, can the sweetness of life be revealed in even the simplest act of a smile.

Alzheimer's Disease is still existing, still encasing minds and destroying lives. But it's leaving survivors in its wake. This is the story of four such survivors. In the end, plain and heartbreaking, love was there, all the way through.

Contents

PART I

Summer 1991, Summer 1998

- 1 -

PART II

Summer 1998 – Fall 2000

- 33 -

PART III

Summer 2000 – Summer 2002

- 89 -

PART IV

Fall 2002 – Summer 2004

- 197 -

PART I

Summer 1991, Summer 1998

Chapter 1

Sometimes, I can't remember. A sentence fades and I stutter. Sometimes I lift my hand to my brow and I swallow slowly. I clear my throat. Sometimes I fear it is my turn.

When I forget the words and the string of phrases don't connect, I remember the stages of his decline and imagine my fate. Am *I* now to be trapped within its web?

THERE WAS AN empty seat beside me, between my mother and I on our flight to Italy that summer we buried him.

"They have screens!" Nicole exclaimed as she approached our seats with her pink, yellow and teal rolling bag. Her hair fell over her face as she tried to lift her bag above her and into the overhead compartment. It was semi light, semi heavy, holding her CDs, extra pairs of clothing, books and shoes. I went to Nicole and helped to lift it up into the compartment. As I made my way back to my seat, my mother winced beside me. I watched her reach beneath the seat adjusting and readjusting a piece of Egyptian blue luggage. It was smaller than Nicole's bag, but with the same sort of wheels on the bottom and a similar black handle on top. My mother didn't want to put it up above us, but rather, have it stay where she could keep her eye on it, to make sure it remained unmoving and unharmed.

We all leaned our heads back against our seats and breathed a collective sigh of relief. We were finally going there, back to where he was born, back to where he had come from. In the years that we began to lose him to early onset Alzheimer's disease, my sisters, my mother and I watched the man with young breath still in him become translucent and quiet. And we knew this town, his and my mother's Pacentro, was where he would come to rest. Maybe it was where we would all finally take a moment to rest. Perhaps, it was I who needed that finality. I had of course traveled alongside him in my own pits and falls and yet I had emerged unscathed, a changed woman.

We remained seated, quietly awaiting lift off. Finally, as I was nearing sleep, I felt the acceleration of the plane and upon opening my eyes, I caught a glimpse of my mother as she made the sign of the cross, praying silently as she tensed before muttering Amen.

Nicole was waiting patiently for the moment when the flight attendant would turn on the headsets and screens, allowing the excited passengers to begin their seven-hour stretch of movies, TV and video games. I could remember what it was like to fly when I was Nicole's age of thirteen. All I had to be excited about were earaches and boredom, perhaps a few pages of a book I'd have a few moments of patience to read in between waiting anxiously to watch a film on a screen I could only see a few inches of. At twenty years old, I felt so old watching her use the handset, watching her know already without ever seeing it before, all the keys to use, all the choices she had. If Flavia were on the flight with us, she too would have been astounded watching Nicole. Maybe she would have even been irritated at the technology and the waste of money gone into this flight. Her frugality was much like our father's. She had been living in Italy for nearly a year, working for Boeing, at the age of twenty-four. We would see her once we reached Pacentro.

I watched my mother's eyes flutter, setting softly, opening slowly. Her deep brown hair hung limply to her chin that seemed to slacken. Her thin lips parted slightly as her brown eyes seemed to draw downwards in sleep. Nicole had already begun flipping through the channels. I took a book out and my mother closed her eyes, finally taking a minute to sleep, perhaps, to dream. For a time I watched her.

WHEN I WAS a young girl, I looked up to meet my parents' eyes, to grab a hold of my father's hand, and fit myself snugly in between them. I wanted their attention on me, their love mostly for me, and I went to great lengths to keep their focus on me.

It started with my coughing fits that made me sweat, that shook my body, trembling small and petite as I lay in bed between my mother and my father. I was nine years old and we were living in Wayne, New Jersey. I had started to experiment with love and the limits I could push, absorb and overcome.

One morning, I awoke with a cough and soon kept coughing. I would pause, taking breaths and staring ahead, enjoying the attention and never wanting to stop. I didn't know that I was exaggerating my coughs, forcing them out, louder and more continuous whenever my parents were near. Only Flavia, who was thirteen at the time, and my cousin Mario, who was eleven, seemed to know exactly what the cause was behind my cough.

One afternoon, when my parents were gone, Flavia and Mario were in charge of me. My mother had told Flavia to take special care of me, giving me medicine if I should start coughing uncontrollably again, giving me soup if I should feel hungry. Flavia must have rolled her eyes during my mother's instructions; her worry must have angered Flavia. Because when they left, and I lay on the couch, watching cartoons in my midday pajamas and resting longer and longer between each cough, Flavia and Mario ran into the living room yelling, "Ok Faker! Who am I? Guess!!" And then they'd cough. Or they'd pretend to be sneezing—"uh—Uh—FAKER!" And it'd end with that word—faker. I'd cry and scream at them to stop but they wouldn't and eventually I'd run upstairs, yelling at them again that I wasn't faking. Slamming my door shut and locking it, I could still hear them with their taunting as I cried atop my bed, waiting for my parents to come back home and make them stop.

Inevitably, that night and many nights afterwards, I'd find myself between my mother and my father, lying down with them on my bed as I coughed and coughed into the night. "Stefania, lay down, calm down, Stefania," my mother would stroke my head, and hold me as my father lay on the other side of me. They'd both take turns rubbing my back, peeling the hair that clung to my forehead, damp from all my energy and sweat. They'd continue voicing their concern to one another; my mother telling my father, "Giovann—maybe we should take her to the hospital." He didn't respond to her but looked at me and held me tighter, more firmly, as though he didn't want to even consider the possibility that my illness warranted such actions. He was frightened at the possibility that my illness was serious, worried at the possibility that I wouldn't get better.

Instead, I was excited by the thought of going to the hospital. I craved validation for the illusion that I had fostered for weeks. And it did happen—one night, I arrived at my new room. It had a single bed, a bathroom, an IV. I jumped into bed and I smiled to myself, hearing my mother and father in the hallway, murmuring to one another before coming inside. "Ok, Stefania. Don't be scared. We gotta go, and daddy has to go on a business trip—but I will see you tomorrow morning, ok? Dammi un bacino, Stefa," my mother told me as she tucked me in. My father stood near me and watched me quietly. I knew my father felt bad leaving me. He often traveled for work. He would travel for a couple of weeks, then come home, leave again for a week, then home again. I was used to it by then—had grown accustomed to my father leaving on trips that lasted weeks, home for fewer and gone again. Maybe that's why I always tried my hardest to be his comrade at home, his friend, his partner.

My mother gave me a kiss and then my father reached down to me. He looked at me and I could see the worry in his eyes, could see his brow wrinkle, his eyes, forlorn. I would grow to know that face, that certain moment where he'd look at me worried and tearful, asking me if I were all right, to try and be strong, pleading with me to fight. And I would one day come to do the same pleading for him.

That night, I went to sleep and most likely slept soundly. A few days passed and while my mother sat beside me, watching a small television that we had rented, my Zio Mario and Zia Franca and their youngest son Mario arrived, bringing with them Flavia and Nicole. My mother was, by this time, worn and heavy with thoughts that plagued her concerning me and my mysterious illness. I didn't think to consider her heavy heart as she stood by me—I didn't think to dream of my father far away, calling me from across the world to hear his hospital-bound daughter cough meekly into the other line. I hadn't realized anything really. I just couldn't seem to fathom the connection between love and hurt, love and guilt, and love and loss.

Zia Franca came in the loudest. She had large teeth and eyes and she bleached her hair blond. She had a patronizing tone, but her firm love was indeed intoxicating. Her husband, Zio Mario, had a bulbous nose and like his and my father's mother, deep-set brown eyes. His hair was graying and he wore glasses to read. He always seemed to keep those glasses somehow glued to his face. I always imagine him with his glasses gripping the sides of his face, up near his temples, so his lenses hugged his chin. His upper lip curved often in dismay and he was never one for hugging. Unlike my father, my Zio Mario often had unkempt hair, though it was much thicker than my father's on top. His hands were large and scarred, dry and cracking; they scratched my cheeks as he methodically went to stroke them. He asked me how I was, looking doubtful.

My sisters came to my bedside; Flavia telling me stories of what she had been doing during the day, asking me how I felt, telling me, in a way, that she missed me. And Nicole walked around the room, touching objects she didn't know the names of and beginning phrases she couldn't finish. My mother told me she would return, that she had to leave but that she loved me and would come back soon. We all shared a moment to say goodbye and then I was left with only Zio Mario, who took a chair by my bedside and sat in silence for a moment. We were alone in my lamplit hospital room and I don't remember any words we may have shared except the fact that I felt uneasy. I didn't like the way he looked at me, the distance between each word, the way he swallowed so loudly as he'd lean back against his chair. Somehow he seemed to entrance me and my coughing lessened without my realizing and when my mother came in after an hour or so away, he got up quickly, shaking his head, "she hardly coughed once when you were gone. As soon as she heard you in the hall, she started again." I watched him leave soon after, realizing my new haven had been ruined.

I stayed a total of a week in the hospital and left a day before I was to undergo a surgery. I suppose it could have been a lie. But my family never mentioned a word—we were happy once more to be together. To be well.

Beside me, Nicole was watching her screen, still enraptured, still enchanted, by all the options she had to choose from. She sat in a black t-shirt marketed for one of her favorite movies, her light jeans straight-legged and tight. Her chestnut brown hair sat shoulder length and falsely straightened behind her ears. She had woken up earlier than she had to that morning we left for the airport, to straighten her hair with her coveted CHI, even if just for a seven-hour flight on an airplane. She had braces, light skin that matched more the palm of my hand than the skin atop it. Her converse sneakers were scuffed and gray from wear. She looked toughened on the outside, but her cheeks were always a bit pink, and her fingers were soft, her nails long and her eyes light. She smiled often, though she wore heavy eyeliner. But she wore her makeup as an accessory to her outfit, as a style. She still ended some phrases on a high note in both tune and tone and she still acted as a little kid would—kind, curious and faithful. I watched Nicole, how she entertained herself quietly, enjoying herself, enjoying the ride, enjoying the many ways to occupy her time. Maybe it was her age or maybe it was something telling about her—but she seemed to favor distraction over sleep, would choose it no matter where she found herself.

My mom had repositioned herself so that her body lay over the empty seat between us, her feet in my lap, her head on a small white pillow that lay against the armrest. She was softly snoring through her throat: a soft nasal streaming in and out. Her mouth was open slightly, showing the top of her teeth. She had light olive skin like

Nicole, though my mother's was a bit whiter, perhaps just more pale. Her deep brown hair was coarse like Nicole's, and her nails seemed naturally healthy and long like Nicole's. I seemed to get my anger from her; in fact, I seemed to get most of my emotions from my mother, my quickness to change moods. I would say I also got her nose—the rounded tip at the end, the slanted tendency of our nostrils.

I was glad to see my mother sleeping, happy to see her taking this time for herself. I had nothing to keep me amused, so I too shut my eyes and tried to sleep. I don't remember what it is I dreamt of on the plane that day—if I even dreamt at all. I don't remember what movies my sister was watching beside me as I settled into my seat, repositioning myself beneath the weight of my mother's feet. But I do know that it was much easier to relax in the air than on the ground. That I found sleeping in the air much easier than on the ground seemed something quite reminiscent of my dad and starkly in contrast to the me who used to fly beside him. I'd have my hands squeezing either side of my head, squeezing shut my ears, as I would desperately try to make them feel less excruciating.

"Daddy! They won't stop hurting!! I hate this! I hate this!!" I'd cry and scream, never really caring if others on the plane heard me, if Flavia was in the background somewhere, rolling her eyes again and thinking, most likely, that I was overreacting. Maybe I was—through my screaming and my crying, my pantomiming moans and flailing arms, yes, maybe I was a bit dramatic. But I can still remember how badly they did indeed hurt. Back when I was young—six maybe seven, eight and nine.

"Look, like this. Just blow." That was my dad's favorite advice to me during those moments of torture. He'd put his face right up to mine, hold his nose with his hand, puffing out his cheeks and sealing his lips, the black hairs of his mustache covering small areas of his lips as he'd take a deep breath and blow. His eyes would squint and his whole face would turn from deep olive to red. For me, the thought of even trying to emulate him was the same if not worse than the pain I already felt.

I never once took his advice and would continue to cry until my mom would interject, "Stefania, teh' mamma, take this piece of gum and chew! Just keep chewing it," she'd tell me. And I'd listen. To her I'd listen, of course—she wasn't the one staring at me, red faced and seemingly about to explode.

We traveled a lot during those early years. I can remember going to Mexico during summers, during short stints throughout the year to differing towns, small and large. I remember sitting in the backseats of rental cars, my father telling Flavia, me, and my mother, "It never rains in Cuernavaca" as we'd near the town beneath the gray and heaving clouds. I can still see that white feather fly into the air, landing at my father's hand as he controlled the stick shift of a rented white punch buggy near Cozumel that afternoon we ran over a chicken on an empty road outlined by sugar canes.

My dad worked in sales at General Electric and we often went to Mexico City because my dad had another office there though he was based in Pennsylvania. In Pennsylvania, I remember always missing him, seeing him sparingly, mostly only seeing and depending on my mother. We had moved to Erie, Pennsylvania from Houston, Texas, where I was born. I was four when we moved to Erie in 1988 and we stayed there until I was eight years old.

I would come to remember the soft sounds of the kitchen, the gentle buzzing of the refrigerator—ice cubes freezing, falling every so often into the bin inside. The tiles on the floor, I would recall, were kept clean and bleached without food or crumble. Nicole would be somewhere close by in her rocking chair, resting and reaching towards her mouth with a toy beside her. Flavia, at her wise age of ten, would be at a friend's house or in the TV room watching *You Can't Do That On Television* or the like. Mom would be in and out of the kitchen, watching Nicole, watching me, cleaning, cooking, talking on the phone in Italian or Pacentrano, the dialect of Pacentro.

There was a calendar we kept on the refrigerator door and I'd count the days and weeks—"Ma, when's daddy coming home?" I'd turn and ask her as she'd pass by me quickly, worrying about one thing and trying to complete another.

"Next week—he'll be back next week," she'd say, as I'd turn to try and catch her eye before she walked away into another room. I'd turn back to the calendar, count the days as my shoulders would hunch over and my head would drop.

But he would eventually return. And I could always see it in his face. His eyes, how they changed when he returned. How tired they seemed and alone he seemed to be until greeting us.

One year, he was gone for my sixth birthday. All that morning I spent alone with my mother sprawled out beside her in their king-size bed. Her door was open just a crack and I heard him walking heavily up the stairs, brushing something loudly against the walls.

I looked at my mother and saw her smile slyly, her eyes at the corners, crow's feet and all, and then I saw him. He stood at the doorway as I ran to him and leapt into his arms.

The surprise of that day was not just his return, but another special someone who awaited me as my father hinted, "Go look what I got you—It's on your bed."

It was Donald Duck—a Donald Duck piñata the size of me, the breadth of two, and everything I could have ever thought I wanted.

"I sat in the airplane and had an empty seat just for him! I carried him the whole way from Mexico City!" He told me later, smiling, proud. It wasn't as though I had a special affinity for Donald; I really never thought of him at all except the times my father would emulate his voice from somewhere in his throat whenever a small child was near. But I kept that duck until the paper feathers turned gray, until one of his arms fell off and his eyes peeled away. It wasn't until many years later that I'd finally have to part with him.

My dad liked to joke about how he was often mistaken for a Mexican man or a Middle Eastern man. His passport pictures dating back to the seventies have pictures of him with heavy beards, mustaches, and with a distant yet piercing gaze. I'm sure it must have angered him to have to pause longer than others whose skin was less olive, whose hair was less black, and eyes less brown. His nose was slim and straight, narrowed and symmetrical like Flavia's. His height was unassuming, maybe even a little on the shorter than normal side. He definitely looked so very Italian compared to the men who would stand tall and towering, white and ash blond beside him and all around him. He loved traveling and working in Mexico City, perhaps because he resembled many men he'd walk among, and he understood their lives and their language better than the culture he adopted when he was twelve.

Because this is a man whose native tongue was for the most part silenced outside his home when he immigrated to America as a young boy. For it was plainly seen in his shoes with even soles and from his steps that sounded a bit smoother upon the streets paved in cement. And behind each step, the distance lengthened between himself and the ancient cobblestones of his childhood.

He was born in Pacentro, Italy—a small town in the mountains, where dwelt a castle and stone and centuries of lives lived and died, and he had this ancient town as his hometown. But when he was six years old, the youngest of two sisters and one brother, he and his family moved to Venezuela for four years awaiting a visa from his older brother, Mario. He must have kept his humor and wits about him though, and must have made the most of it. In our living room, I often pass by a framed photograph of him enlarged in black and white. It's a photo of him and his classmates, for what seems a costume party. He's around nine years old and sits in the front row dressed as a cowboy—how fitting. He's the only one who looks away, rolling his eyes up towards his classmate to his side, playfully holding up his gun and thumbing his belt loop with his other hand. Everyone else just seems content enough smiling straight forward towards the camera.

At twelve, my dad and his family finally made their way to Patterson, New Jersey. And that year, my dad found himself in his first American grammar school. He came to school a Giovanni one morning, and left that afternoon as John, having been forced by the nuns to Americanize himself somehow so that others would accept him. Thus began his new life in America—but his new name didn't change his spirit.

"Stefa, I worked two jobs throughout college—and I left with six thousand dollars saved," he told me on numerous occasions, emphasizing the fact that he always knew the value of money, of keeping it and saving it—while focusing on ways to keep earning it. One of those jobs he had in college was at a bakery in Patterson, where he worked nights, making and filling donuts. And on one night, alone in the shop, he cut his hand on the donut-filling machine and managed to fill a number of donuts with jelly, or with *pink* custard—a blend specific to my dad, made of course, with his very own blood.

He never seemed to shed that newness of him living in America, especially not after marrying my mother, another Pacentrana whom he met one day in the Piazza Iaringhi on one of his returns to Pacentro when he was twenty-eight years old. Ever the confident and outspoken lady, when she was twenty years old, she saw him, the Americano who visited his friends, his aunts, his uncles, in Pacentro every now and then. She recognized him that afternoon in the square as she yelled to him, "Eh, Americano, mi compri delle noccioline?" In my mind, I picture her grinning as she flirted, and him, I see him laughing in response to her asking him to buy her some peanuts—a luxury in that mountain town at the time.

After college he lived abroad in Brazil, Asia and Europe and even New Jersey for a time. He learned six languages from all of his travels. My father graduated with an Electrical Engineering degree and found job after job related to his field and in sales, each job higher and more prestigious than the last. He believed the way to succeed came with sacrifice and with uprooting himself almost constantly. After he and my mother married in Pacentro, not long after he bought her those peanuts, they lived in Chile for about a year, then returned to America, to live again in New Jersey, where my sister Flavia was born. He would decide to leave New Jersey again, to find a better position within GE, and so not long after, they moved to Virginia, then to Texas, had me, stayed a time, and moved to Pennsylvania, where Nicole would be born, where he would try to give us all that spirit of travel when we were all young, favoring Mexico above all other destinations.

I never cared about the sand in my suit or the sunscreen on my nose when I'd sit in front of my dad's legs as my mother rubbed the same sunscreen on his back the afternoons we'd spend at the beach. He squinted his eyes and I'd watch him. Maybe he squinted at the friction of her skin upon his, her strong caressing and attentive ways of making sure his back was protected and his small, round bald spot on his head greased and covered. "Giovanni, credo che stanno crescendo i capelli—" My mom would tell him.

"You think so? I know! That medicine—it *does* make my hair grow!" He would buy bottle after bottle of Mexican-made hair growing formula. At times, my mother tried to make him feel as though it may have indeed been working.

I always found the white streaks on his head amusing and smiled when I'd get close to him asking him if he were ready to come in the ocean with me. He would sit most often in a chair, half of his body blocked by the oversize umbrella, and half would burn beneath the sun—because undoubtedly, he'd have fallen asleep. He'd fall asleep and forget to re-lather because my mother would be the only one to think of protecting him. And I would run back and forth, from the umbrella to the sea, hoping the next time I'd arrive he'd be awake, that he'd motion me over beside him and tell me to take one of his many beach resort baseball caps and set it down beside his shoes as we'd run into the water and dive in.

My mother, I always assumed, would never come. She'd sit on her lounging chair and read, bending her knees and resting a magazine against them. Her large sunglasses covering her eyes, her visor set snuggly on her head. But suddenly, sometimes, she'd surprise us all when she'd decide to get up for a swim and I'd be so happy during those moments. I'd get so excited.

Or sometimes, too, I'd sit beneath the beach umbrella, calling my parents, "Please, please let me buy something!" For as sure as I knew that one brief second of eye contact would lure the men with shiny jewels and linens and toys, so I knew that my dad would give in amidst my mother's objections. My dad would look at me and nod slightly but tell me curtly to wait for him and not be too loud with my choices.

Soon the man I'd summon would sit before me and like a queen I'd look through his treasures. I often paused on the rings, the silver, and pointed to some I liked. Then, my father would sit beside me and start the ritual of bargaining he so loved, loathed, yet loved even more.

He'd raise his voice, but keep it steady. Refuse to buy and turn away, getting up to sit again in his chair. I didn't understand these games he played, the role he assumed when he began to bargain. He controlled the unassuming man much like the strings of the marionette puppets that clinked and swayed from beneath the bundles of objects that this man and others like him, would cling to and display for all the eyes that promised money on the hot and scorching sands.

Finally, after excruciating minutes filled with tense and fluid Spanish, I'd wear my treasure, but with a tired satisfaction and a nearly dashed desire for the piece of something my father had purchased. He was like a boxer, a champion fighter, scouring away the excess numbers associated with his purchase, not following or missing one step against his opponent, the seller, the alleged scam and the sordid attempts at taking advantage of his children, his wallet, and his intellect.

THE AIRPLANE WAS dark; I always thought it sweet yet odd that the flight attendants had the power to shut the lights out and create an environment for sleeping. Did we pay to be treated like children? Or was it a luxury? I guess it's difficult at times to tell what the difference is between the two sorts of treatment. Perhaps, maybe perhaps, it is just difficult for me to discern. It was in a way nice to be taken care of like that, to be tucked in, to be doted over. I certainly hadn't lost that side of me since those years as a child, when I'd hunger for it, search it out and find it. But it was most often, after the storm, after some trying time, that I'd want the attention on me. I hadn't known back then as a child what the power of illness could bring, what power it had. I used what meager means I had to bring a sense of unity, though it was in vain and it was most assuredly selfish in its aims. But what of illness, anyway? Is its one saving grace that it can produce a sense of unity? Of peace?

I think my mom may have noticed me looking at her, re-adjusting myself in the seat, finding my backside a bit numb. "You awake?" She asked and I nodded. She sat up, put her feet down and looked at the handset connected to her armrest. "Want to watch a movie?" She asked.

"Yeah, of course," I told her as we started scanning through the selection and I looked over at Nicole who had fallen asleep herself.

Chapter 2

Pacentro—lying still and quiet amid the Appennini Mountain range in Abruzzo, Italy. When I sit and wonder, imagining myself floating there among the hills, the valleys, the little tunnels and the miles, I imagine the excitement I always feel when seeing the town emerge from behind the shadows and within the crevices, sitting strongly before the distant Maiella Mountains that stand like a fortress far beyond the town.

I see Pacentro a little clearer as I near it in my thoughts, seeing angles more sharply than before as I climb around the roads covered in white pebbles and dust, outlined in weeds and bushes that grasp at the narrow road that winds itself upwards.

Yet my earliest memory of visiting the town must be when I was seven, my legs swinging against the seat of our rented four-door. I sat next to my father as he drove, accelerating around and around the road that hugs the edge of the side of the town on the Monte Morrone.

There are two ways to ascend to the town, and that year we drove the route against the hunchback arc of the trees that still hang drowsily over the curved angles of the road. Those same trees must have felt the changing winds year after year as time lent itself to more treacherous ways of ascending in fast cars and motorcycles, competing with a mixture of speed and fear along the sharp turns of the road that lead up and down Pacentro. The road leads up farther still, up to where the road to the cemetery bends right before the canopy of coniferous trees that shelter the small and timid heads of the wildflowers. On the other side of town, climbing steadily up the gradual slope of the mountain, another road turns and falls, but less sharply and abruptly, and the views of the Appennini melt within the air, the land and the wind. The times I've ridden in the backseat with my sisters, or later with my cousins and friends, are the moments that have awakened another vision of the town and its limitless side. These glimpses of the gradual becoming of Pacentro are the images that seep inside my mother, as she'd tell me again each year, sitting in our backyards in America, "Stefa, when I sit outside, and the wind moves my hair, against my cheeks—and the wind in the branches, I think of Pacentro. I imagine the mountains and the birds that fly in the air around them—I miss Pacentro, Stefa, those mountains—they follow me wherever I go."

That year we drove up the turns while listening to Nicole's Disney Music mix tape on repeat. My father drove steadily and I peeked in the rearview window, catching glimpses of my mother looking down at Nicole, who at one-and-a-half years old, slept soundly near her bosom. Eleven-year-old Flavia sat quietly beside our mother, staring intently out the window beneath the perm of her hair and skinny frame.

It was the first time I remember visiting Pacentro, the excitement breathing into me as I spotted the town from below—the whiteness of the buildings, the contrast of the light against the dark hills that surrounded the town and the small homes that speckled the valley around it. I remember the shadows of the trees we drove beneath across my face as I tried to manage my childlike urgency of seeing, of touching, of being in that town that seemed to beckon us forward as we made that initial ascent.

I try to imagine if we passed the cemetery that afternoon we entered the main square—the Piazza Iaringhi—whether or not we drove slowly upon Via Del Convento into the bustling center of town. We may have entered from the other road, coming to a quick stop at la Curva just after passing through the street on which my mother lived as a child.

Veering left, la Curva leads to Il Girone, a small park where stands a stone statue of La Madonnina, or The Virgin Mary, set against a backdrop of the Valle Peligna and the sprawling town of Sulmona. Opposite the statue is the slope of the Monte Morrone. There, drivers speed quickly by in their cars, eyeing spectators or ignoring them entirely as they make their way up the mountain looking for a view, a silent getaway, a drink in the restaurant that stands farther upwards on that road.

To the right, la Curva leads to the Piazza Iaringhi, the town's center square, and to the small fountain set against the wall of a building, where in the afternoons, old men stand against it, smoking, talking, and children bend their heads slightly, dangerously straddling the wet stone with their shoes.

What I do remember is sitting beside my father as he parked his car in front of a brick wall. I recognized nothing.

I remember stepping out into a sun that beat down on me from a land I never knew to really be my own—except for the traces that lay within my breathing, within my name from both my mother and my father. We walked out of the car and into greetings from old women who stood beside us and voices yelling, "Benvenuti! Ma come siete cresciuti." The women in their aprons and their flip flops and slippers and children who resembled me in their brown hair and tanned skin, their look of long unknown connections they kept inside their faces as they stood on balconies looking down at us, walking slowly around us and standing quite near us. And finally, what I do remember is entering his house that afternoon we arrived in Pacentro.

My father's home stood on a narrow street, a few houses down from a stone-backed spigot that spilled forth crisp water from the melted snow of the peaks of the Maiella Mountains you could see if you stared towards the sunset. The front door was wooden and heavy, laden with small cracks and deep grooves. It held a rectangular lock in the center, a keyhole and small lever you pushed downwards as the key turned inside the lock. And after hearing it catch, the door would creak open and inside you'd stand upon cold and whitened stone flooring.

Before he left Pacentro when he was six years old, my father lived in this home. He would run down the stairs, pass his mother in the kitchen before slamming the door shut behind him. Maybe he'd settle on the cracked and barren stoop where I would later find myself on afternoons. I spent many hours on that stoop, often accompanied by Nicole, who ran along the small pathway between the doorways that often stood ajar, with only their beaded streams of brown or colored beaded curtains to block out the heat from the day. I'd often sit outside where I could hear the language my parents shared, the language of the town, the small language inside my own head that I couldn't always understand. I'd bask in the recognition and the understanding I felt for the familiar smells in the kitchens around me, the yells, the screams from children, from mothers.

There was a boy my age who wore the same shirt day after day. It was light blue with a picture of the characters from *The Simpsons* in the center. To complement his shirt he wore the same blue, gray and black shorts. The day he finally changed those shorts was a day my family noticed gleefully—"Mom! Fernando changed today!! He has pink and black pants on now!!" Flavia was the first to notice. She was older and often left the house in the morning, returning for lunch before leaving yet again. We all shared in the excitement that day he changed his pants—though it would be temporary.

I saw all of this as I sat on the stoop, capturing moths as they landed amidst the powdery residue of the surrounding gray stonewalls. I would sit and wait for their flittering, flapping wings to land peacefully for a moment before me and then I'd lunge at them. Squealing in joy, I'd cup my hands around them. I'd try my hardest not to start to panic when I'd feel their wings like eyelashes tickle the insides of my palms as I'd lift them away from the walls they'd try in vain to mask themselves against. And then, after a moment, I'd let them go again, as I'd wipe their dust against my jeans and sit and wait once more.

Several years later, after we moved into our new home in Chesterfield, Missouri, we would swat similar moths with brooms as they flew, panicked, hitting themselves against the corners of the off-white walls in our hallway. Whenever my sisters or I saw them, we always called to our father to exterminate these unwanted guests. I never questioned the need to kill them until the night my mother told us that we shouldn't—that they were most likely our reincarnated relatives. Perhaps, she said as she pointed to a moth my father nearly had cornered with his broom, perhaps that one was his father, Papa Alberto. I was hit hard by her words, begging my father to please, let him go, let him fly away. But my father resisted, continuing to bat at all the moths beneath the yellow tint of the hallway light.

WE TOOK A small tour of his old home that day we first arrived. We set our luggage in the living room across the kitchen. His mother, Nonna Concetta, still owned the house and she lent it out to her children, her nephews and nieces, to anyone in the family who requested as long as the time slot was available. The house had been painted and renovated with new appliances, a renovated kitchen and eating area. Though the structure was for the most part the same, the same staircase and bedrooms. We walked up the stairs that first day and I peeked into a bedroom as my parents and a woman who led us inside made their way to the other bedroom and the balcony. I laid my book bag down in that bedroom where the whitened sheets lay cleaned and a breeze blew in from the window, the lace curtain rising and falling with the air's breathing. I then followed the sounds of my family out onto the balcony, its edges guarded by a black iron railing, and basked in the view of the town and the Appennini. Where we stood was on the northern tip of town, so that the majority of Pacentro lay sprawled before us, to our left side. In our family room, we keep a picture of my mother and father soon after marriage: my mother still glowing in her wedding gown and my father still grinning in his suit. They are leaning over these same rails, holding one another's hand, beaming.

Once inside, we passed by the bedrooms again and my father turned to us. He stopped by the room where my book bag sat sideways and told us, "I was born in that room." I was elated and astounded. I felt compelled to keep that room forever—keep it as a memento, a family heirloom, forever.

"Really?" Flavia, too, was enchanted and my mother stood smiling. Another part of me tried to imagine Nonna Concetta as a pregnant woman, as a younger woman, rearing my father and watching him grow. I couldn't imagine too much of her besides what a sour and short woman she was. She had dark brown hair like ours, though it was lighter than her son's, my father's. She had deep-set eyes and wrinkles all around them and down her cheeks—they traced her neck down to her chest. She wore black daily, though at times I could see a hint of her white lace underneath. Her husband, my Papa Alberto, had died just a couple of years before that trip and she kept with the tradition of mourning. My mother used to tell me that when I was one and two years old during our visits to their home in Patterson, he would chew grapes in his mouth that he grew in his yard. Then, he'd put those same chewed-up grapes right inside my mouth, feeding them to me amidst my mother's screams in protest. He was my father's father.

Nonna Concetta's stockings were thick and nude colored—the type that old ladies usually wear. I couldn't see a blemish on her legs because those stockings were so opaque and thick. And her shoes were black, often heeled slightly. She wobbled a bit when she walked, slightly to the left, slightly to the right. And her voice sounded strained, seemed complaining even in a "Ciao" and in a kiss. Nonna Concetta's spirit seemed tough if not spiteful and she had a look in her eye that always seemed to be seeing something distasteful. I never quite had a conversation with her except a few smiles here and there and a kiss I'd bestow regrettably on her cheeks when my mother and father told me to.

Yet she had been young once and had worn her own apron and house shoes around that home she once kept. And as much as I tried to imagine her as a young woman in that bedroom, nestling her newborn son, I saw only what her life had left her: scarred, withered and embittered. Yet my father must have seen his mother in her for I will never forget the way he doted on her, sometimes looking at her with those same big eyes and that mischievous smile as though he were about to tickle her or break into his favored Donald Duck sounds. And Nonna Concetta, she would smile at him and smirk, one of the few times I'd see her face contort in such a way that was sweet, docile and motherly.

I would spend that first summer sleeping in that room, in his birth room, and finding out bits and pieces of the past that would create a small haven of memory I will so desperately cling to in the years to come.

MY FATHER AND I left the house one afternoon to visit two of his cousins. I didn't recognize their names, nor could I keep them in my head as we made our way towards the spigot. "Stefania, try that water—it's so good—try it," he urged me. I managed to soak the front of my shirt. With my bangs dampened and stuck to my forehead, I tasted the cold water as it flooded my mouth, mimicking what he must have done time and time again as a young boy running with his friends, pausing just a moment for a mouthful of water before continuing his play.

We turned away and soon entered a much larger street, Via San Marco, which leads to the large Piazza Iaringhi. On this road, homes built atop one another and apartments clad in century-old brick and mortar lie on either side. Old women sit on small wooden chairs outside their open doorways, talking loudly to one another and stopping briefly to stare at passersby. Old men sit with their chins resting in their palms alone on their balconies in white undershirts and heavy five o'clock shadows. My father and I walked hand-in-hand along the road, stopping every few paces to greet a relative or a friend. He would introduce me and I'd kiss them on either cheek, wait for my father to nod a promise to visit and grant a temporary "Ciao" and we'd be on our way again.

When we neared a large tunnel that opened up towards several steps, my father stopped. "Stefania, see down there?" We looked through the tunnel and I remember seeing more heavy stones that matched the street and walls reddened with cracked dirt and enlivened with bugs. "My aunt used to live there, just at the bottom of the steps. That's where we're going—to see her kids."

I looked up at him as he stared down that tunnel. I caught a glint of light from the afternoon sun reflected in his dark brown eyes. "One day when I was young, younger than you, I was running down those stairs with my friend. I tripped and fell and hurt myself—I bled so much. That's how I got this scar on my chin."

He lifted up his head and ran his fingers over the small indentation that lay atop the crevice of his cleft. The scar looked to be only a centimeter long. I had never noticed it before.

That summer, I managed to steal many moments with my family, with my father. Yet the only memory I retained with such clarity and detail besides the moments I remember of boredom, of fighting, of moments all twisted around one another, turning into one another— the only memory I cling to of that summer was of my father falling.

Chapter 3

Her headphones were hanging atop the tangle of wires, her shoulders holding them up close to her ears. I watched as Nicole's head slowly dropped more and more towards me, her body shifting against her armrest, attempting to sit semi-horizontal on her chair. I always hated having her lean her head on my shoulder when we'd be in the car driving together—my mother in the passenger seat beside my father driving, Flavia on the other side of Nicole, and me bearing the brunt of Nicole's sleep. She would still be young, still shorter than me and I would still be too young to know how mean I could be.

But I was older that day on the flight, I had endured much that had caused me much more discomfort—I had caused much more discomfort for her, the least I could do was offer her a shoulder. I tore a blanket from my lap and set it upon her. And my mother—she had commenced snoring soundly, softly and gutturally. I could hear it even if I tried to drown it out with headphones, with sleep, with my heavy thoughts that I knew must have clouded my ears that day.

And then the plane would shake with turbulent winds breaking the line ahead of us and we all felt it.

As a child, I didn't pay much attention to turbulence. I was much too concerned with my ears—my father, with sleep, Flavia with a book, with "The Babysitter's Club" or the like, and my mother, with reading, with praying, and yes, a bit of sleep as well. Nicole, I don't remember too much of within the plane rides. I just see her as a baby when we all traveled together often. I don't remember her as a preteen flying with us all during the years my feet didn't touch the ground, didn't rub against the luggage beneath the seat in front of me.

And maybe it is I don't recall being bothered as a child by turbulence, by the fearful dips and turns because maybe I had plenty at home. Maybe those alarming moments of panic and fear and confusion were evident in those versions of love my parents exhibited for themselves and for us. The fighting seemed at its peak just eight years after the summer I first slept in his room, catching moths in my small hands and imagining him falling. Eight years later when he was forty-eight years old, he was still falling, my father, faster and more severely this time as he answered the phone call that afternoon telling him he had the brain of an eighty-five year old man. It was the same year Nonna Concetta died, nine months earlier, from dementia and diabetes. She was eighty-one.

My mother was the first person to suspect Nonna Concetta could have dementia after she had traveled to New Jersey to help care for her after a surgery and noticed the oddities and the inconsistencies in her behavior. She grew sickened seeing her maxi pads, used and soiled, lying on the bathroom floor. Drying, according to Nonna Concetta, in order to be used again. And my mother tried to tell my father's brother and sisters, Zio Mario, Zia Emma and Zia Lina. Yet no one had believed her, calling her, instead, a liar.

Perhaps even my father shrank away from her with disbelief because his mind was already fading, and again my mother was the first to notice the changes.

"I could tell with the tips—at restaurants. He would hold the pen unsteady in his hands. I'd tell him, 'Giovan—che stia fa?' and he'd get mad and then he'd write something and I'd have to take it away from him and do the math."

We never did eat out much because of my father's preoccupation with numbers, with money, with maintaining his financial nest he intended for himself and my mother after retirement. He would remind our backyard neighbors and closest family friends, Linda and Nick Rallo, over and again about the importance of keeping a cushion for something, something that may or may not happen, a cushion for the fall.

But around late 1996 and into 1997, my mom started keeping a list in her mind of all of the things that didn't quite seem right—and she'd notice first, the pauses, the moments he'd clear his throat, his hand clenching tightly to the pen as it danced around the check while he'd think and plan what he needed to write.

I think perhaps he noticed it too—as he'd sequester himself in his basement office for hours on weekends, reading in his mustard-yellow leather chair, pointing to sentences he'd find in books, ideas he'd read and try to share with me. There'd be self-help books of all kinds—*Learn to Speak Better—More Confidently, Improve Your Memory Now*, and others. I would often hand him espressos that my mother would make for him and try quickly to leave before he'd start attempting to teach me what was in those books—trying to address the fact of how it was so important to start early—but I never wanted to listen.

I seem to recall that my father remained as such even after that phone call that afternoon. He was thinking, perhaps, that maybe he could find a way to stave off his impending dementia.

Yet my mother kept finding more and more differences in her husband—that confident man she met in the square years before in Pacentro. She even feared he had lost interest in her and that he didn't love her anymore.

It's difficult to see my mother as a woman yearning after my father, trying to cling to him as he grew distant. But this distance was not what my mother feared, it was something else entirely—something a simple question of attraction couldn't seem to answer.

There were many people, his doctors included, who blamed depression. Depression often causes forgetfulness, a loss of interest, a loss of passion, of will. And what seemed to be lacking in my father only grew more noticeable to my mother. Surely it was more than depression, she'd think to herself, as her list would get longer. And she kept that running list until it flittered in her own hands, tearing in her tightened and desperate grasp.

BUT IT WAS imperative to either one or even both my parents that we plan another trip back to Pacentro. Thus we returned again, seven years later, in 1998, when I was fourteen, Flavia, eighteen, and Nicole, seven. When I imagine myself that summer in Pacentro, I cannot remember the ascent into the town—only the arrival. We chose to stay in a rented apartment much closer to the Piazza Iaringhi, off a small side road just a few hundred meters long. The home was built upwards, floor after floor of beds and bathrooms. That summer I had shed my shorts and tranquil musings on the stoop and chose instead to sit inside and read, listen to Flavia's walkman when she wasn't around, and try and amuse my father, who seemed tired, worn and sad most of the time. And I worried each time he and my mother argued, worried that she might race up the stairs into an empty room. I feared the fights would escalate like they did one afternoon that January when Nonna Concetta came to visit.

My mother hadn't wanted her there, not after everything she had done for her and the nothing she got in return. Not after warning the family about her dementia and receiving no faith in return. Flavia and I were upstairs, getting dressed hurriedly as we heard our mother's familiar shrieking and screaming that came from the depths of her. They fought often—but that January the fight was heightened and we knew this one would most likely end in hitting, in my father banging his head angrily against a wall and my mother breaking anything she could lift.

Nicole was at Flavia's bedroom door the afternoon we tried to make her come with us—"Nicole, please, it's not good for you to stay here when they're like this. Come with us—we'll go see a movie," Flavia pleaded with her. But she just stood with a certain aloofness that comes from habit and shook her head as she headed for the basement to watch television.

Flavia and I decided to leave her there. We left and we laughed and we drove for hours and then, when we came home, no one was there. Our backyard neighbor Linda had left a message on our answering machine to meet at her house so we left our kitchen, with paper and chairs strewn on the floor, and walked through our backyard and into hers and there we found Nicole playing with Linda's daughter, Nathalie. We saw Nonna Concetta walking around Linda's house, wandering, mumbling against Linda's blond hair and white painted walls and framed pictures of her family and memories too happy to forget.

"They were arrested—your parents. Enida got scared and called the police when your dad kicked her and then the police came—they took them both." I remember Linda telling me, her soft and gentle smile falling at the corners, and her light and docile voice appeasing my questions and my need to know what happened and why. Afterwards I lay on a flowered chair in Linda's living room. I stared out the window, trying not to let my eyeliner seep into her cushions as I picked lightly on my wrists.

Not long after, they were both released and I stayed with my mother at Linda's house while my father and Nonna Concetta shared ours. That was the first night my mother heard me scream in my sleep.

PACENTRO WAS A haven of sorts that summer—a place to recharge and stay away from the stress and the changes going on in our house. My father still cried a couple of times in the living room in the chair that faced the open window from which we let in the cool mountain air during the evenings. But for the most part, we had distraction. Flavia toured the streets with Nicole, sheltering her from getting lost and protecting her when my mother was at a friend's home getting an espresso, or talking loudly with women in the streets. And I remember the visits to the cemetery and the small inkling of recognition I felt seeing the names on the mausoleum's white stone walls and the pictures that hung below the iron-wrought names.

On the mornings we'd visit the cemetery, we'd first stop at a floral store in the Piazza del Popolo. In the opposite corner of the square stands Pizzeria al Forno, owned by my parents' friends, Franca and her husband, Ernesto. The restaurant acts as a central meeting place for many of the townspeople in the small square. Beside the restaurant, there is a narrow road called Vico Diritto that connects the Piazza del Popolo to the Piazza Iaringhi, where cafes bustle with gossip and jokes and momentary pauses of others contemplating their day. For lifetimes, people have walked steadily upon Vico Diritto beneath the balconies and the empty and taut clotheslines lit by the street lamps mounted to the walls of homes built centuries before.

The Piazza del Popolo is the small piazza that houses the Church of Santa Maria della Misericordia where my parents were baptized and eventually married. The face of the church stands erect and wide, bearing a clock on the right, high beside the upper window. The walls are made of thick stone, water-stained in areas and browning with dirt. Beyond the front of the church looms the bell tower, measuring close in height with the castle towering farther up into the town. In front of the wooden door bordered by an elaborate stone fixture sits the fountain shaped as a sepulcher, where small children crawl and bend beneath as they laugh with one another, sipping water as it spills from spigots bordering the sides. And near the entrance to an older part of town, towards La Guardiola, is the floral shop, and there we would oftentimes buy lilies and carnations and bring them to our relatives in the cemetery.

Once inside the cemetery, to the left stands the building housing my mother's relatives. It is a white building with white steps leading to the second and third levels of an open-air mausoleum. My mother and Nicole would walk hand in hand ahead of us. My dad and I often walked to the trash bin standing on the outside of the stairwell, filled to the brim with empty bleach bottles or unmarked and empty plastic gallon jugs. He'd grab one and I'd do the same, following him a few paces to a black piped faucet which resembled the stone-backed spigot near his childhood home. We'd fill each container with the cold water and walk slowly up the stairs to my mother who stood sweeping and cleaning her parents', grandparents' and great grandparents' corner of the floor.

I'd usually walk around aimlessly during that time my mother would snatch each flower, gracefully tearing away the dead leaves and browning petals, replacing the sour water with the fresh water we'd give to her. I'd look at the different names in the wall and look closely at their faces. I'd think about the years these people lived and when I'd tire of looking at these strangers whose names often matched my own, I'd return to watch my mother dutifully keeping her parent's corner spotless. I'd watch her wipe away the dust that would settle on their pictures and I'd see her kiss her fingers to their names, to her mother's name in particular. My mother's mother, Flavia, had passed away when my mother was sixteen. My mother had been her caregiver for months as she suffered slowly from cancer. Because her father was an abusive alcoholic, my grandmother's death was especially hard on her. After she was gone, my mother was alone except for her younger sisters, a brother she barely spoke to and a father who was bent on making their lives miserable.

Each time my mother would look at her mother's picture, she'd pause a little longer than she would otherwise. She'd make the sign of the cross and pray silently before sweeping one last time and gathering the dead flowers and leaves to dispose of. Nearby, my father, who stood behind her, turned to walk away.

The sunlight from the stairwell reaches into the open doorway of the third floor, and I imagine my father must have squinted his eyes before descending those white stairs. He would have turned to go as my mother stood praying, and I wonder if she held her breath as she turned to him in bed that morning a little more than a year later, when she finally let go of her list she kept of all the ways he was changing. I wonder how he reacted that day she turned to him and asked, "Giovanni—tell me, what's eight minus five?"

And he—"I don't know." I wonder how long she lay beside him and what words the two of them shared before a silence would have fallen so quick and heavy, cold and forceful like that same rush of water that filled our empty gallons in the cemetery.

This of course would have occurred after we returned. After we traveled back home and the weather would have eventually grown frigid. And it was then, finally, that the phone rang that afternoon, as I was most likely in my room, reading magazines or books on witchcraft I had just purchased. I was dabbling in depression, touching merely the surface of feeling emotions I wouldn't know how to handle. And Nicole, with her missing tooth, would have been playing with the neighbors' children again, her glasses sliding down her nose; and Flavia would have been studying in her room, her senior year in high school, pressuring herself to do well and succeed as the phone would have rung and he would have answered.

And that's when it would have all begun—that afternoon when the doctor confirmed what my mother had suspected—my father, at the age of forty-eight, had the brain of an eighty-five-year old man.

PART II

Summer 1998 – Fall 2000

Chapter 4

The night within the airplane changed to morning as the flight attendants began opening up shades and turning off cabin lights. I heard the bustling of the passengers as they awoke from sleep, repositioning themselves in their seats, preparing for their meals. Because Nicole, my mother and I were in a row in the center of the plane, we met the sun on our sides as we stretched and lowered our tray tables, watching the flight attendants approach our aisle.

My mom and sister both still had sleep in their eyes, and their faces still had that lasting impression of exhaustion and momentary moodiness like a child often does upon first waking. We ate in silence, as Nicole continued watching her screen, and my mother and I mainly ate with our eyes downcast, staring down at our food.

When we finished eating, we put our trash and empty plates on the tray table of the vacant seat between my mother and me. It was my mother's idea, as she triumphantly stretched out her legs so sore and tightened from the long journey. I lay back against my headrest once again, and listened to music streaming through my headphones.

If Flavia were on the plane with us, she would have had to take the seat that sat empty, emanating an absence yet a sense of relief and company. Her tanned legs, muscular and athletic, would have stretched far beneath the seat in front of her, though she'd have taken great care not to bother the passenger whose legs she'd avoid hitting. Her fine hair, which had grown much longer than ever before, would hang lightly against her shoulders that would sit tall and rigid, pointy, yet fleshed. And her lips, thin and much like our mother's, would have shut easily as her eyes would have pondered the words she'd read in an Italian novel, or a feel-good story with religious undertones. Those hazel eyes of hers would look at me annoyed as I would try to ask her questions about the book or start a game of how to bother her best, as I'd often do, effortlessly, as a child. But there would be that feeling I often had when around her, that feeling of safety and understanding—that feeling that only comes after you've pushed just far enough to feel the edge beneath your toes, and arrive, quite breathless back again, with two feet planted firmly on the ground.

AND SO IT was back then, in 1998, after my father received that phone call. Though we would yet to feel the ground again beneath his feet, nor would my mother as he hung up and looked at her. He looked at her and told her and remained emotionless if not unworried, as I remained locked in my bedroom, thinking the world lay suffocating all upon me and that it strangled my limbs in all its attempts to flail me.

I was, most assuredly, in my room at the time the phone rang and my father answered. Probably, I was sitting on the floor, my back against my mattress, my books sprawled before me, open notebooks, pens, CD cases and, mainly, me alone with myself. Because that was just how it came to happen that I made a different sort of haven within my bedroom, a space that I would sit within myself and wonder outside my window. I'd sit and stare for hours and feel the waves of my despondency rise and fall, breathing in and exhaling out my fourteen-year-old sadness where now resides words on crumpled papers I have since found stored in my closet—words of poetry that mainly spoke of pain, of sadness, of escaping. Really, the pain I felt during those early years—really, it all originated within me and I never seemed to know why. And for that reason as well, I felt guilt for feeling so sad and for beginning to separate myself so far away from my family and my friends. It seems I made myself a hook inside the ocean, rusting from the rays of the sun ensnaring me; for I too, was beginning to feel the effects of my father's dementia.

Eventually I would come to know these emotions so fully; I would say I knew them all along. But I don't believe that was true during those afternoons in my bedroom. In eighth grade, I really had only myself to blame for everything that originated within me. Each moment I blinked a second of my memories away, those memories that proved there was a time before my depression had set in.

I was most likely listening to loud music, pounding beats of some sort of screaming and heavy drums that drowned out the moment the telephone rang that afternoon. My anger was streaming out from the cracks in my doorway, down the stairs and into their silence.

Hours passed as my parents settled in to watch television that afternoon, most likely the stock market channel, calmly and collectedly watching the numbers and letters flowing fast at the bottom of the screen. The sun would start to set as the hours would unfold and I'd still be sitting in my room, writing poetry and thinking, scratching at my arms and wrists with a needle I had taken from the laundry room. I didn't think much of it, nor did I see the real harm in poking my wrist and getting the needle wedged beneath a layer of skin, running it across my wrist like a bracelet made of pink string. I would sit and imagine myself going deeper, imagine the small beads of blood streaming forth like cold, fresh mountain water, spilling forth from a spigot encased in stone. But my Pacentro was far away and I didn't find it on my wrists back then in my bedroom. I felt lonely—I know. I felt like the only one who had any sense at all.

WHEN FLAVIA STARTED college in September, Nicole wouldn't stop crying. When we left Flavia in her dorm room, Nicole couldn't be consoled. "Fla! I don't want to leave Flavia!!" She cried as we ushered her into the backseat of the car. My mother and father kissed Flavia on the cheek, holding her briefly before turning around again. I waved goodbye from the backseat, missing Flavia's first real absence and tried not to get too irritated with Nicole's wailing. But somehow, Nicole's quivering bottom lip and her eyebrows all drawn up together to a meeting on her forehead always got me—it reminded me of when she was a baby, her tongue hanging midway outside of her mouth and I'd always try to push it back in. Moments like those always seemed to beckon me when I'd be on the threshold of full-blown annoyance with Nicole—yet somehow she always seemed to make me melt in spite of myself. She was the only one I felt guilty with—the only one I'd really try with—well, some of the time at least.

We left Flavia in a town in Illinois about three-and-a-half hours from our home. I remember the phone calls home she'd make, not too long after the first day she watched Nicole crying into my shoulder as we dropped her off. I'd be in the basement and I could hear my mother yelling on the phone, "Flavia—you need to try to stay a little longer. Naggia Sant, Fla, we just took you there—" I hadn't expected Flavia to be so unhappy and wanting desperately to come home. She was always so strong, so individual and happy with herself. I admired that in Flavia, the way she diligently studied for courses, feeling so drawn to excellence, yet still having fun simultaneously. In her bedroom, I often looked through her yearbooks, reading messages from her friends, seeing her in pictures on the pages every so often from the many clubs of which she was a member. And I found it so odd that she could look so happy but still feel so sad.

Flavia was not perfect and she fought often with our parents, most notably during her teenage years. Our father never liked us borrowing from others, which basically meant we couldn't borrow dresses, shirts, or even a skirt. He'd yell and chase us, make us return whatever it was we'd borrowed, and Flavia never quite understood why. Especially that day she was to go to a dance with a boy or on a date I can't remember. I sat in a corner of her bedroom, hearing my father's roars from the living room as Linda tried to console her.

But it must have been the boy inside him, the young Giovanni who came through Ellis Island at twelve years old, learning a new language and a new name that made it quite impossible for him to suspect his family was in need of anything he could not provide.

That night Flavia cried into the phone, my mother reassured her that our father would be driving there to see her en route to Decatur, Illinois, or various other towns he'd frequent on business.

And it did come to happen—he did take her out on lunches and small talks. Flavia never quite told me about them at the time, but later, she would recall, "When I would cry and tell him I wanted to come home, he'd say 'okay, come with me, you can just go to SLU.'"

He was trying to help her no doubt, but Flavia knew that that was something he would have never said before. That something was changing or had changed hit Flavia hard during those lunches. Where was that man who never gave in to failure or fear, that man who challenged Flavia all those years? I can see her sitting across from him in a restaurant during lunch, her eyes readjusting their focus on his face that probably seemed placid as he ate big bites of food. He would tell her not to worry, downplay her move to college and the time of her life that he had strived for in blood at donut shops and language barriers, the only child in his family to go to school. He never settled with us, made things easy for us. He believed in making us see the challenges he faced growing up and make us feel the same pride and consternation when faced with weakness as he did those days he'd chase us up the stairs swearing he'd kill us if we wore a friend's dress.

"I guess that's when I knew he was maybe a little sick," she told me recently over the phone when I asked her about those times he'd visit.

How was it that from that mere suggestion, Flavia knew it was true? She probably had other clues she kept together in a section in her mind, like my mother. She and my father used to run together. Flavia and Dad. They'd sweat and grow red in the face and love every second. I would wait for them at home with a pen in my hand or the remote control beside me while they bonded over running. I tried, once, to wedge myself inside their moment, but it didn't stick and I much rather preferred my tournaments with him at the foosball table in the basement, our games we shared since buying the table when I was eight years old. Yet, Flavia again noticed a change when he stopped being able to run with her the whole way. When he'd grow tired, she'd wonder why but keep going. She may have looked back at him as he'd come to a stop. But she wouldn't look for too long. She just kept going—kept going until those lunches when she finally let herself realize why.

I have since tormented myself for taking so long to figure out the signs I first saw. I often think about what it is that caused me to blanket myself in my own emotion. Of course, I wasn't blind to his forgetting things or seeing his personality change. Instead, I remember pushing it all away as I seemed to focus more on the shallow ways of dress I hid beneath, the black laces around my wrists and neck, my hair I'd dye black to match my eyes, and I remember again that perhaps I did just swallow it all whole, all of the changes and the moments that warped and bent my heart.

I'm sure that after those lunches when Flavia would swallow, hesitantly pausing after each word my changing father said, I'm sure she must have struggled to keep her wall secure from doubts. She was always the one to be able to muster such strength. When I asked Flavia to continue telling me more about those lunches, a bit more about that day jogging when he fell behind, she tells me she can't remember. So it's me who must fill in the gaps and imagine her face as she spotted him stopping, as she listened to him talking. It's me who must remember for her. I guess I owe her that, can recognize that—I am at fault. But why? Because of those moments I kept to myself and the ways I hurt myself while all the while he was falling.

"But I never believed it—or wanted to believe it. That he was sick. I blocked it out and really, when I would cry it was mainly because of you—because you were so messed up. I was so worried about you, not dad. I didn't want to believe he was sick."

One year at Christmas, she took our silent family dinner and decided to quickly fill the air with nature sounds—with baaing sheep. Nicole's eyes lit up as she watched her oldest sister suddenly spring up out of her chair and race out of the living room doorway and right smack into the credenza. She lay moaning later on the couch, bleeding from her nose, amidst the sound of her sheep.

Flavia's random acts of spontaneity were moments of pleasure for all of us. Those moments were used as a means of distraction for us during those silent meals when our changing dynamics were the only true thing we had. So we thrived on the little awkward times, the funny moments—we savored them, much like Nicole, who never seemed to remove her eyes from the screen on the seat in front of her. Nicole reminded me a lot of Flavia—her strength, her ability to switch focus. Both she and Flavia proved up to the challenge of laughing, of smiling—of carrying on while I stumbled behind. They were there though, waiting for me, holding their hands out to me. But for the moment that year, I didn't bother to reach my own hands out to theirs.

Chapter 5

In the cemetery of Pacentro, there are two main mausoleums—La Cappella del Rosario and La Cappella di San Carlo. There are also many smaller Cappelline with the names of the families who own them—families who can afford such extravagant, private chapels. Yet, the majority of the Pacentrani are buried within one of the two main Cappelline. This practice is based on a tradition originating over a century ago, where each family belongs to a specific confraternity. My mother's family is housed in the Cappella del Rosario—her family members being a part of the confraternity of the Virgin Mary of the Rosary. My father's family dwells within the three-story building of the Cappella di San Carlo, the confraternity of Saint Carlo Borromeo.

In 2000, my father again descended the stairs of La Cappella del Rosario on an afternoon my mother brought flowers to her family. His eyes squinted against the white marble stairs of the two-story building as he walked towards the Cappella di San Carlo. I caught up to meet him, our shoes crunching against the dirt and small stones, beside the buzzing of the wasps and the flies that paid their own type of homage in the air. We passed beside the small fountain where once we had filled two plastic gallon jugs we had scrounged from the trash bin. We walked ahead of my sisters who stood inside with my mother, looking at names and thinking of our relatives we had never met before. And my father and I—we walked among the pinecones that had fallen from the trees that lined the way to the Capella di San Carlo, across benches lining the edge of the pathway. We walked as one beside the small wall made of darkened stones cemented together in rough design, that borders the path on one side, while on the other, trees and small, private mausoleums align the edges of the cemetery. We veered left, up the few stairs to a gated building—protection from the wild boars who often roam the lamp-lit burials in search of water, of food—of the flowers that must smell like food to these beasts.

We kept going straight, down the opposite set of stairs and around the building to an open ceiling, with squared plots positioned in columns up and down the walls. Each plot had a face staring outwards, just like in my mother's building—each face of a life lived and gone, now ghosts who inhabit the hearts and memories of the people who knew them once. Their names, the dates of their births and their deaths are written in iron, and a small electric lamp is mounted below the dates.

My father led me to some of his family members, his cousins, his aunts. Afterwards, he led me to a different corner, to a man who shared the same name as him, but whose plot had no dates and carried no picture. It was an empty cement square with just his chiseled name: "Giovanni Silvestri." He was set apart from the newer graves in a corridor much darker than the area of the center. And in this darkness, my father brought a flower to set inside the vase mounted beside his name and smiled. I'm sure it was fear of ending up like him—a name with no past and no future—though more likely for him, it may have also been a sort of friendship, an understanding, a curious fascination with a man whose life was left unnumbered but whose name was made to stay.

As a child, I'd always just follow his smile, the way it swept across his mouth so lightly; and I always kept a lighthearted gait as I followed him around the graves. And soon after, we'd leave, passing the small hallway made of white stone and mortar and exit the iron gates to that pathway lined with evergreens leading up into the town.

A year prior, my mother had purchased her grandfather's house, the home in which her mother had been born. It sits in the older part of town, La Guardiola. The entrance to La Guardiola is located just past the floral shop in the Piazza del Popolo, up the street from the main church. There, you walk down a small cemented hill and turn left at a small statue of the Virgin Mary. The pathway turns to ashen cement, looking centuries old and feeling quite uneven, making walking a bit difficult, though if you pound upon the ground you surely would feel the strength of it—the thickness, the assurance of its foundation. Walking further downwards, seemingly ancient stone homes with windows shut in with heavy curtains, and voices weaving in and out of buildings that seem to have been abandoned. The cracks in the surfaces of the walls seem startling, yet they look more like life lines, wrinkles in the skin of this street. At one point, the path leads you to an archway, with a small, stone bench reaching upwards from the ground. Once outside of it, the wind from the right catches your attention towards the ledge leading you straight to our home. Outside, two women usually sit beside one another on chairs they dragged from inside their cantinas. Maria and Giuseppina—two women connected to that home of ours, like the paint on our shutters, the screen of our window in the kitchen, the light spilling in from outside.

Once inside, the house begets a home as the sounds of our voices, our feet against the tile fill the dark and lonely crevices of the rooms. Upstairs, my sisters and I share a bedroom. It is located directly beside our parents' room. Both rooms possess a large window, behind two glass doors that latch together with a gold-colored handle. When I open those doors, I release the screen that catches at the bottom of the window, letting it fly upwards, careful not to let it catch within its frame. One more obstacle before I clear the window—the green blinds that rattle against the window, sounding like tin beating against the wall.

And then the balcony—and the mountains, the way the air flows like silk against my skin. My hair lifts and falls from the passionate wind that greets me and I feel the beauty; it greets me, the same as every year I return.

The floor of the balcony is paved and grooved—the rough surface scratches the bottom of my feet as I make my way towards the black iron railing. To my right is a small, roofed room meant for storage, and the plastic ceiling rattles just like the blinds on the window. To my left is a sink against the wall of the balcony facing the houses and homes that sprawl the mountain towards the western side of town. And ahead of me, summoning me all around me, is the view of the Appennini Mountain range, the Maiella in the distant east, and my breath that catches in its wake.

That summer would have been the first time I set foot on the balcony and stood against that railing, watching the swallows dive down towards the tops of the homes that stand silently below. And then the background would come into focus and those same birds would be just specks of dust in the sky as I'd stare into a mountain opposite me as it stood pulsating before me.

In an area that could be considered its heart stood a large boulder with its face painted in green, white and red. I tried to imagine just how large that face must be—tried to imagine my hand, spread out upon the red, my pinky falling into the white—tried to see the sweat, hear the quickened pulses of heartbeats and breaths as that was the place, the starting ground, for the annual Corsa degli Zingari. This race is an annual celebration, a tradition commemorating the apparition of the Virgin Mary, who desired a church be made in her honor. Each year, men and boys born in Pacentro line up against the stone, shoeless and fearless, and then run down the jagged slope, their feet pummeling against thorns and branches, sharp rocks, and stumbling into small creeks. And as they'd reach the valley, I can imagine their determination pushing them onwards as they'd run swiftly through screaming cheers and familiar faces and up towards the outskirts of the town, right into the small church, La Chiesa della Madonna di Loreto, with the bloodied path of debris left behind on their feet.

But that afternoon was months away from the race, which happens every September. I had never even watched the spectacle—but he had. He had stood time and time again with his family, his cousins he'd meet again each year on visits to Pacentro from America, from Poland, from Korea—from wherever he may have been living and working at the time. I saw a picture once, he in bell-bottomed pants, chin-length sideburns and shining eyes standing beside his cousin as the runners made their way across the valley and onto the road leading up the mountain. I see him in my mind as I try to recreate those moments where the mountain comes alive. I try to hear his laugh, join in his cries and envision a man I saw then depleting now in front of me.

That summer, I hardly ever left that balcony. In every angle of the sun, I sat with my legs dangling between the spaces of the railing, the grainy cement leaving grooves on my legs. On sunny days, I'd lay a towel down and sunbathe while listening to music, my sunglasses catching beads of sweat as it poured from my head and down my temples. And before I knew it, I'd find myself cooling off as the sun began to set. I'd sit with my back against the glass storage room, letting my eyes trace the edges of the mountain, outlining the shapes of all the houses before me and below me.

Sitting on that balcony became a way for me to unearth myself from the weight of home and of him—from everything up until that point that lay upon my own emotions, mixing into me, forming me into a pensive, solemn person. Much like he had now started to become. Quiet, unsure of himself and slipping. Outside that balcony, no one really noticed or really believed anything truly was the matter. I knew it—my mother did. My sisters. And we carried it with us when we traveled there that summer, waiting for my mother to decide whether or not she wanted to move back, return to this town, this mountain town, to live.

She still hadn't decided if she was capable of taking care of him all on her own. Because she knew the ending before it ever really began. Yet everyone else beyond that balcony had only assumed that he was just depressed. And the me who sat against the glass wall and in the arms of the town, surely must have shaken her sixteen-year-old head and, looking up into the sky, felt the remnants of the years before—back in 1998 when a smaller version of herself first realized the numbers were leaving him faster than the sun now set.

I had laid my hands on my dad's shoulders, asking him to go with me to rent a movie. I was face to face with his bald spot which he always said he knew the way to cure. But those times he traveled to Mexico and stopped at the pharmacy to get his "miracle cure" hadn't seemed to have done much to give him back some of his hair. He always seemed to think some was coming through though. And we always smiled and pretended that it was.

Annoyed, he told me to wait a second, as he spoke softly under his breath, a mumbled expression in Italian to show his frustration. But he gave in after my continued prodding—my moment of excitement that he hadn't seen in a while. I was fourteen years old and was just beginning to wear black. It was the year I was only just beginning to learn how to forge a smile.

After choosing our video, he laid it before the cashier and waited.

"Name and address, please," the woman said, as she looked up at my father. I glanced down at him as he scavenged in his wallet, clearing his throat. I returned my gaze to the woman, who was also waiting, nearly staring.

I watched him flip through cards and pictures in his wallet, finally pulling out his license and handing it to the woman. She seemed satisfied and typed something into the computer, then asked for his phone number. And again, he cleared his throat.

"Um. It's uh, it's—wait a second." He clenched his jaw; his hands trembled slightly as he opened and closed his wallet. He finally put his hand to his forehead, and looked at me.

"555-3937." I told the woman our phone number and then turn to my dad. He wasn't watching, rather, but gazing down towards the counter.

Afterwards, we hurriedly walked towards the car. I put my seatbelt on as his hung beside his tense body. He fumbled with the keys as he tried to start the ignition.

By the time we pulled up to the driveway and parked, he had calmed down. I got out of the car before him. I stood in front of the garage door, tightly grasping the video in my hand, looking down at my feet, at the cracks in the driveway, at the invasive moss growing in between.

My father was near my side in an instant and flipped up the cover of the gray and plastic garage code opener. Before he had a chance to punch in a number, the cover fell back down onto the number pad.

He cleared his throat, and raised the cover up again.

I watched him move his finger across the numbers, adjusting his glasses, rubbing his eyes.

"One more try," I thought before giving in to myself and his sullen eyes and reaching forward and typing in the code. We walked inside together, looking down at our feet.

SEVERAL MONTHS LATER, three days before Thanksgiving, my father answered the phone and was told he had the brain of an eighty-five-year-old man. He looked at my mother as he stood motionless, if not indifferently. I can almost see the panic in my mother's eyes as she watched him hang up the phone, telling her the news, and then perhaps just walking away. I can almost sense the fear rise into her body, the panic, the terror.

Pacentro became locked in her mind—the people of the town became a hopeful source of aid that she knew she'd have to utilize if her husband's health did not improve. And so when she learned of a house that had previously belonged to her grandparents (and had later been bought by a couple from Rome), was now up for sale, she bought it—she bought the house not just believing it would be a summer home. This was now one year after that phone call, when she'd lain awake in bed, planning out a return to a town she had left when she married my father.

But there was still much in between—still much had happened to push her to buy a house, expecting to return to live and leave America behind.

Instead, the doctors revealed later, after my mother had called them back wanting to know why they didn't ask to speak to her instead, that maybe my father was born that way, that perhaps he had had a brain of an eighty-five-year old man his entire life. How could the cells be dying? They had asked themselves. He was just forty-eight years old. Surely, there must be another explanation.

But my mother knew. And so she took what means she could to try and salvage his brain as best she could. A few weeks passed and my mother decided to buy a watch for him—an expensive watch that he had never had the heart to buy for himself. It could have been a token of love and fear put together, one last test before turning back towards her list. And in the very beginning, he seemed to love it. But when he was asked to use it, he'd only be able to respond, "the big one is on the 4 and the little one is on the 6." And so, my mother realized finally, she had bought him the watch too late. It was already happening and nothing could turn it back now. Not even tricks to stop it.

"OK DADDY, THIS one. 5 + 8." Her small fingers grasped onto the crisp, white flashcards. I never noticed how large they seemed in a child's hands as Nicole, at seven years old, showed our dad another. I had just come downstairs into the kitchen and walked in on our dad's warm-up—his "brush-up" on math. My mom had just bought some elementary flashcards for my dad to practice. Nicole, not yet old enough to know all of the answers herself, still took some time along with daddy to guess.

I put my book bag on a chair at the kitchen table across from where they sat side by side. Nicole had lost a front tooth and her pink wire glasses framed her face in a soft, angelic and childlike manner. Her shoulder-length hair resembled her hair on the plane that day, and again her look was honest and hopeful.

"Nic—why are you doing this?" I asked, annoyed as she sat fiddling with the flashcard in her right hand, while our dad sat with his shoulders hunched and heavy.

"Mommy told me to, Stef," she said, agitating my father, who seemed to start in protest, trying to end our fight before it began.

Looking back, I don't believe now that I really saw the tragedy of the situation—I'm sure I felt it, I must have felt it as I mumbled,

"Whatever," trying hard to mask the stutters of my father and Nicole's encouragements as I opened the cabinet and reached for a pot.

As I waited for my rice to cook, setting it down to simmer, I walked to the living room with my pants sweeping behind me, and sat on the green leather recliner sitting adjacent to where my mom lay on the couch. She was staring, entranced by the television speaking quickly in Italian. I let the words wash over me, not listening yet trying in vain to hear something, anything, other than Nicole's small voice in the kitchen.

"Stefania, what the hell are you wearing?" My mom asked, looking down at my splintered jeans and up to my black shirt, beneath my black cardigan, down to my wrists adorned in shoelaces and lace.

"Ma, stop," I told her firmly and defiantly. Each day she asked me. I had dyed my hair black again and she had yelled, but later accepted it—telling me I seemed more Italian—if I'd wear less eyeliner, I'd even look normal.

I smirk now remembering how right she was, though how I questioned the idea of normal. How I pushed the idea to the extreme thinking no one understood—no one possibly could have known what I felt like underneath all of my disguises.

And hours may have passed before our first fight. I most likely spoke without thinking, or yelled at my mother for asking me to do her a favor. I may have said something, cursed at them; I don't remember exactly. In any case, a fight ensued and my father would have helped to lessen the screaming or punished me, slapping me, shaking me—if my mother did not do it first. I surely did deserve it—their aggressive ways of managing me, the palms of their hands against me. They brought their ways of raising me from the painted boulder to the Church and finally, into our home in Chesterfield, Missouri.

And minutes would have passed before I would have heard Nicole tapping on my door, whispering into the cracks. "Stef? Let me in, Stef. Come on." I'd be sitting on my floor, my eyes puffy and my anger thrilling silently around me as I'd search for some way to calm myself. And in my mind, I see the same scene happen again and again, and really all I can remember is the aftermath: me sitting against the soft cushion of my bed, my Salvation Army knife glistening red and sitting still, and staring deeply within my newest wound, all the while ignoring Nicole outside my door.

I TURNED AWAY from that paint-covered boulder and back into the window, shutting the green blinds against the glass doors and locking them. The shadow fell against my body as I left the sun behind the white curtains, following the faint sounds of my father's fading voice.

Chapter 6

In December of 1998, about a month after the phone call, my mom took my father to another neurologist. It was the day she would first learn of the three-question test, a screening exam for supposed sufferers of dementia. My mother remembers vividly the moments of the exam and how they terrified her, making her know for certain—and with medical evidence to back her—that finally there was no turning back.

My mother and father sat for the first time in a private room with a neurologist who administered the test. The doctor would ask him a color to remember, a number to remember and a thing. Ten minutes later, he'd ask the same questions. I assume my father thought of the three-question test much like an eye exam—fuzzy answers to questions that seemed to change even if no lenses were before him. And a blank stare would ensue, a few stutters and prideful attempts and then, finally, a shrug.

After the results of this exam, the neurologist was the first to clearly believe with conviction that my father had dementia. He would refer my parents to Washington University for further testing the following month.

So it was that my father's fancy titanium watch got put in a drawer in the credenza in the kitchen. Just a few weeks after buying the first watch in December or January 1999, my mother bought him a digital watch. That same month, they made the short trip into the city to Washington University. Housed within that university was the Alzheimer's Research Center and various neurologists roaming the hallways in lab coats and glasses.

There they were both interviewed separately. My mother recalls: "For three hours, I had to talk about each and every moment since the early 90's when your father and I fought, when he acted weird, when I started noticing changes."

Simultaneously, in another room, my father sat with another doctor and a nurse. He answered the questions diligently though I know neither how he did nor what he did and said. If he twiddled his thumbs, how many times he may have cleared his throat—if he indeed knew any of the answers at all. I can only imagine the outline of his jaw clenching tightly during each pause.

Surprisingly, the doctors simply labeled his condition a "syndrome" without any hint at dementia. They gave my father prescriptions for antidepressants and a referral to a psychiatrist. Perhaps he was just depressed.

My parents left and drove home as I was sneaking a cigarette outside, reveling in time alone and knowing nothing of what passed between the hours they had spent away from home that day.

INEVITABLY, MY FATHER was fired in September. I hadn't suspected that could happen to my father—that he could fail, that he could let himself fail. But I didn't know he hadn't *let* himself—he had tried his hardest to simply remain afloat. Yet it did come to happen. The months before, he had taken his antidepressants dutifully. If it were true, what his doctors had inferred that January, the pills would have been enough.

And I didn't have a clue that he was suffering at work. I watched him in the mornings getting ready to leave; I saw the light beneath the crack in the doorway of my parent's bathroom. But after that night he didn't come home for dinner—well, that was it, was all it took really, for me at least, to realize something had changed.

My mother and I were waiting for him in the living room. Nicole was in the basement and Flavia in Illinois. And my father was sweating at his desk in his office, hearing the clicking of the clock on his desk, feeling each light in his coworkers' rooms go out and their footsteps walking quickly towards the exit. And he, I'm sure his fingers were shaking as he swore in Italian over and again, "Cazzo—naggia la mis—'" starting phrases and cutting himself off. Tearing off his glasses, rubbing his eyes and breathing in strongly through his nose, feeling his chest tighten as he stood up and pounded his desk with his fist.

"Ma—should I call him?" I asked her, looking at the time that neared 9:30 p.m.

"No—no he'll come. Let's wait a little bit." She retained her calm and I don't understand how she managed it. Perhaps she wanted him to struggle and test himself, see if he could still work on his own without our worry or concern—without our help. She wanted to see if he could still manage on his own. Sort of like watching a child struggle to stand, she wanted to see if he still could.

And he—I can see him in my mind, his face taut with anger and frustration at his computer screen that failed to act as he wanted. "Everything seems broken," he surely must have thought.

And while driving that night, I'm sure he must have taken fast turns and forgotten to signal; he must have run a light or two and scared another driving beside him.

"He's home," I remember thinking as I heard the garage door slowly creaking open and his car door slam. I went into the kitchen and watched him walk inside, grasping his briefcase at his side as he began tearing off his jacket.

"Stefa—can you help me with this thing I have to write?" he asked, and I sat down beside him without answering.

"I started to write it—and it did something and the whole god-damn thing got erased. It took me hours," he said as he propped the laptop open and handed me a sheet of paper with about a fourth of the page typed.

"This took him hours?" I thought to myself as I looked at the paper, typing, looking over at him as he sat fumbling through another stack of papers that he had set in front of him. After minutes, I was finished.

"Dad—I'm done. Do you want me to help you with something else?" I asked.

"What! Already? Naggia Cristo—I spent five hours doing this. No. No, I'm ok. Just go!" He was angry but I knew he wasn't at me. He was frustrated and he was livid and he stayed in the kitchen working, or rearranging papers on the table, until my mother and I went up to sleep. I still heard him in a chair every so often pushing it out from beneath him, the legs scratching away at the tiles. The pressure of his body and the force of it as he'd stand and reach for another document he probably didn't understand in the end, echoed inside my head as I lay awake that night in bed.

But where was I really—what was I really worrying about—as I'd lie awake in my room? I can write now, looking back on that girl who cried alone in her bedroom during the weeks her depression was at its strongest. The version of me who read books on Satanism, witchcraft, searching for a sentence that would make sense, grasping me with its claws, the meaning slicing into me, awakening me. I can see my heavy melancholy striking me over a friendship lost or a relationship failed or simply from the feeling that no one really could understand me. Like ash, I drift across my head, watching my cutting get deeper and my disregard for hiding the wounds get sloppy. But all of that seems secondary the moment I suddenly hear the volume of the television grow louder as he settles down in the recliner. He sits down in the green recliner, his final destination for the day. It is perhaps just a few weeks before he is to be fired. He no longer spends his weekends preparing for the week. He leaves his desk a jumble of notes, of scribbles and scratches in pen across papers creased and stained by old coffee.

The way he'd sit on that chair was always the same. He would bend his arm, rest his hand against his head and move again, sitting still with his hands in his lap. His digital watch would beep every hour or so and I wonder if he'd glance at it despondently, not understanding what it was that made him feel so hopeless.

And upstairs, his feelings seemed to match my own, though our reasons surely differed. In fact, back then I really believed my feelings just sprang from nothing—nothing really, at all. Besides the fact that I couldn't get along with anyone, that my depression lay thick and heavy on my senses and that I couldn't find a way to see through it. My depression was my sickness that seemed to mimic the same sickness I had as the young girl of my memory. She still seemed to live inside me, and the power of sickness seemed still to live a life of its own. It had now evolved into a darker illness all over my skin, and downstairs it seemed to punish him the hardest.

IN THE SUMMER, a month before we left for Italy, I got a job working at a movie theatre just minutes away from our home. I would slam the car door shut after my mother dropped me off and run my black nails through my hair as I entered in through the doors. I never cared much for small talk with my coworkers who all stood a bit away from me, not understanding my pallid face or my moments of humor that would come spilling out from my mouth in times when I would find a release from myself. The day a boy I worked with told me, "Your new haircut makes you look like Trent Reznor," was a day I felt so proud—proud to look like my favorite singer at the time; though he was a man, he was an artist. On breaks, I would smoke cigarettes outside beside my coworkers—choking on nerves and anticipation; I was always a bit unsure of myself but sure as ever that I wanted and needed the moments of reprieve that a cigarette would allow me.

And then they would come on afternoons and sometimes evenings—my mother in front of my father who stood nodding to people around him in his large framed glasses, his polo shirt tucked into his jeans. He was beginning to feel freer with my mom and it was no doubt nearing the time when he'd be let go at work. Maybe he was already pulling out all the plugs in his office, maybe already knowing where he was headed.

"Stefa—we came in for free! I love that you work here—you can never quit!" My mother would joke, as they'd approach my line at the concession stand. I'd turn around to fill a large soda for the both of them—fill a large bag of popcorn for the two of them. And my dad would snort that lovely snort of his as he'd laugh, the snort that originated towards the back of his nasal passage, in his mouth, back towards his throat. I do the same when I laugh now, laughing a bit longer and feeling a small pang knowing we laugh the same. And better yet, when I laugh a bit harder, my seal-like laughter escapes from me and it's my mother coming through so that in times of joy and in jest, I feel the two of them, see the both of them, jovial and alive.

Because he had been fired, my mother had panicked knowing his bosses and his coworkers had no idea what was happening inside her husband's mind. She was able to get the necessary documents together in order to prove my father's disability, and so he didn't get fired after all. As a result, he kept his insurance, his pension, his everything we needed, intact. He was to be put on medical leave while my mother made appointments with other doctors, most notably a renowned neurologist named Dr. Holtzman, though he couldn't see my father until the following January—January 13, 2000. Time was not wasted as my mother filled the months in between with three other neurologists—all left unnamed as their diagnoses all spoke the same. In unison I can hear them all as they face my mother and my father in an office, degrees hanging sharply across the walls, books in shelves behind them as they calmly set their pens beside their folders. "Dementia" they all would say in unison. "Dementia" my mother would repeat. "Dementia" they would say again, firmly this time, and that'd be the end.

My mother became my father's voice as he lost his own. His pride she knew she needed to keep intact. She was the starch in his clothes she ironed that he wore day after day on that green recliner, and the crisp fold of his collar in March of that year, 1999, when my father, Nicole and I went to visit the Rallos.

It was more than obvious to both of our families that the Rallos had become my parents' closest friends in Chesterfield where we lived cattycorner, one behind the other. It's difficult to say whose house was actually in front of the other—whose was first and then the other. All I know is that the ground grew muddy and our shoes squished in the wet grass of our neighbors when we'd make the journey to one another's homes. In winter, the ground would be littered with our footsteps, when the snow was not too deep. And in summer, we'd bend the blades of the dry and yellowed grass, hearing the crunch of the branches beneath our family's willow tree.

He wore a belt and jeans and his college ring from Farleigh Dickinson on his right hand, his wedding ring on his left. His stomach did not protrude far as he still jogged most mornings, coming home sweating and fatigued asking me or someone to pour him a large cup full of ice, filled to the brim with a mixture of orange juice and water, telling me all the while that I really should start exercising. "Look at me—it helps. It makes me feel good," he'd say while I'd laugh, knowing how much I hated running and how I would never come to love it as much as he and Flavia seemed to love it.

"Hi John!!" Linda Rallo exclaimed upon opening the door and seeing us. The light from outside sparkled off her blond bob and fair skin as Nicole passed by her, running inside before us to find Nathalie. "I'll get Nicholas, he's in the crib in the living room," she said. My father and I stood in the hallway as Linda came back with Nicholas in her arms, wrapped in a white blanket, in an off-white nightgown. She set him in my father's arms and for a moment my dad just looked down at him, at Nicholas's sleeping eyes and the way he lay lax and relaxed. A smile etched upon my father's face as he looked down at this baby with the softest of eyes glistening, while his hands held him with such strength—yet still so tenderly. Nicholas lay quietly within my father's arms. The two seemed bonded together, seemed connected.

We often shared dinners with the Rallos—family get togethers were always open to us. And they learned a great deal about my father's fascination with the stock market and financial security—a cushion, as he'd come to call it. He pressured them to do the same years before and would grow annoyed and angry when he'd see them spend their money fitfully, according to his tastes and his sensibilities. And when, after returning home from visiting Nicholas, my father would return to the stock market, to the basement where he'd frequent his online portfolio, selling and trading throughout the day—he didn't suspect that he was, for the first time, causing more harm than good.

"He would sell and buy all these stocks that didn't make sense. He didn't know what he was doing anymore and I would yell at him to stop," my mother later told me. She had learned the trade from him back in the days when he'd receive his Barron's magazines and study them from his fluorescent lamp light in the basement. Those days, just a couple years before, he'd tell me excitedly how he was going to multiply his earnings each year, making millions, by following the same trading principles and subsequent successes he had developed. But my mom stopped him before he managed to slide miserably down a path of financial ruin. She hoisted herself into his seat in front of the computer in the basement and began to fix his mistakes.

THE RALLOS WERE the closest we had to family, and they began to learn of my parents' shifting roles. Linda would receive scared and frantic calls from my mother. Tall and inviting, Nick would try to entertain us, bringing us together with his sharp wit and kindness. The family was a mixture of American and Italian American members, an amalgam of traits that seemed to do nothing but complement one another. Nathalie, their oldest child, had wavy light-brown hair; Sophia, the youngest, freckles and a red head, and newly christened Nicholas, a blue-eyed boy of smiles. And they all seemed to love us in return—they all loved my father; he was their friend. I knew this well and believed in it because this family believed our family when everyone else seemed to disregard my mother's fears entirely.

It's strange to think that in a moment you can realize how alone you are. In a moment you can realize that the idea of family is organic—everchanging and variable. So my mother thought as she stared into the telephone in March of 2000, dialing the number of my father's brother—that Zio Mario of my childhood. It had been about six years since he spitefully touched my cheek with his dry and coarse hands. My mother assumed as she dialed his number that Zio Mario and his wife would without question embrace the idea that my father was unwell. Though they had not been speaking for about a year because of issues from the past, my mother believed perhaps she could still reach Zio Mario regardless.

She sat, my mother, on our floral-carpeted steps. Her face so swollen with gray bags beneath her eyes as she opened her pink phone number book, searching for Mario Silvestri.

"Hi Mario, it's Enida—" she started. "Mario, you know Giovanni has not been feeling well . . . I took him finally to a neurologist who thinks that he might have Pick's disease or Alzheimer's disease. He wants to know if you and your sisters will donate blood to do research—"

"How dare you call me? You only call when you need something! I am OK. Lina is OK—Emma. We're all fine. How can you say these things?"

"Mario—" she continued, until her voice turned into a sob she tried hard to stifle.

It would seem that Zio Mario would have naturally responded in earnest, attempting to believe her. But he and his wife looked the other way and shunned the message in the call altogether. They didn't show a sign of support or believe her. Instead, not long afterwards, the rest of my father's extended family even accused my mother of making my father crazy, of making him depressed. It was my mother's fault, and it was all a lie.

Chapter 7

Zio Marco had come to pick up me, my mother, my father and Nicole at the airport in Rome in the summer of 2000. I stepped out of my Zio Marco's van with sunglasses on and my baggy jeans covering my shoes and squinted as I looked around the near-desolate Piazza del Popolo.

When my family and I visit Pacentro in the summers, Zio Marco is always the one to pick us up in a rented van. He stands in the airport with his arm bent at his side and his palm against his hip. When we see him, he kisses us once on either cheek, hugs us and turns us back away in a hurry. Just like my mother, he seems always to be thinking ahead, pressured in some way for time. Marco is a man who murmurs words, raising his voice every now and then when speaking to another or when something passionate awakens within him. He sits solemnly in the evenings in a white undershirt, his heavy arms resting on the kitchen table as he stares ahead of him. His thinning hair glistens beneath the light in his kitchen; his thick mustache sits unmoving on his tired face as his wife, Franca, bustles around the kitchen, feeding him pasta and bread.

That year I was sixteen and I'm sure it must have puzzled him to see my eyes hitting the ground. Yet more likely it didn't. To my side, Nicole, much taller at the demanding age of nine, was smiling beneath the sun. Nearby, my dad still seemed to hold a strong gait and smiled confidently and spoke somewhat fluidly, though his voice was quieter than usual and he seemed to have much less to say than in prior years. And my mother—perhaps if he cared much at the time, Zio Marco would have seen a hint of the fear that lay inside her. My mother is Marco's younger sister and resembles him in the deep brown of his hair and the way his eyes seem to lie deep within his face, creating a darkened tint of skin below them. But even in the moments when her back is bent to its extreme, her sanguine nature rises to the surface and she stands with her eyes unwavering.

It had been three years since we last traveled to Italy. And in that time, not much had changed—except us. I guess that's where the attraction lay in medieval towns that garnish the mountains. Perhaps that is where the comfort lay. For my mother—I would assume that's what prompted her to first think of returning to live in Pacentro and buy that home down Via Guardiola.

It was about a three-hour drive to Pacentro from Rome. I stared out my window, my headphones nearly shaking from the volume of my music as my uncle parked his van outside the small flower shop beside the bend of the road we would take.

"Stefa—grab that bag and help Nicole—" my mother told me as we stood beneath the stares from the villagers on their balconies. Without a word, Zio Marco led us down the twisting path, past the voices and the smells of lunch that filtered through the screened windows and open doors. And when we reached our door—that's when we first saw Giuseppina and Maria. Giuseppina in her late eighties, sitting on a wooden house chair, bending forward, leaning her elbows on her lap, chewing something invisible in her mouth and squinting around the sun to see inside our faces. She must have heard that we were arriving that day—she must have been ready for us. My mom greeted her quickly—"Giuseppina—Ciao! Ma, com'a' sti?" she said as she bent towards her, kissing her on either cheek.

"E, Mari'!" my mom started, turning to Giuseppina's side, towards a woman who jumped from her chair, embracing my mother tightly then, in turn, my father and us. Maria was the mother of my mother's childhood friend. Her eyes were round, lively and kind and she seemed in every way the opposite of her friend Giuseppina, who sat hunched in her chair, uninterested. Maria's hair glistened white and she still had her teeth, which didn't rattle in her mouth as much as Giuseppina's seemed to jangle like ice in an empty glass.

My greeting was less enthusiastic as I shrank from the questions and mandatory answers—how old was I, what did I study in school, did I behave? A simple stare seemed to ensue when my answers were given curtly, if not unwelcomingly. I was tired and didn't feel like pretending. I was already so winded by their hugs and their language that I just couldn't find an ounce of me that was willing to speak.

When I entered the house, I remember feeling the warmth waft through the windows my uncle opened hastily. I can still see the shadows sprawled across the wood paneling on the walls and the stone-tiled flooring in the kitchen set apart from the living area. Outside the kitchen was a cement step set against the front of the house, supporting the backsides of neighbors who sat beneath our kitchen window. "E! Giovann!" I could hear the women yell as I made my way into the darkened living room. I heard his answers in mumbles and then I heard them laugh. He was making those women feel at ease with his jokes and his kindness, making our entrance into their quiet street welcome.

Inside, my father may have walked up the stairs soon after, following the sounds of my mother as she left the women outside to begin unpacking in their bedroom. "No, Giovanni. Leave me alone. Go downstairs with Stefania," I can imagine her tell him as he approached her. He was not unlike a small puppy searching for love from his master—a toddler seeking to emulate his mother. "Giovanni—stop!" she snapped at him, as he fumbled in the suitcase, touching clothes, attempting to do—something. I imagine him feeling useless, walking out onto the balcony, standing completely still and listening. And I see the reflection of the mountains in his glasses as I see him in my mind, absorbing the scent of the wild brush and earth, the air bathed in rivulets. I wonder what it was he might have thought standing there, looking at that town he left behind so many years ago as a child. My father—did he think he was really getting sick? Was he considering coming back—was it only really based on my mother's decision—did he have a say in that at all? But I don't think he thought that far ahead—no, I don't believe he saw much in front of him but the sky, the green shrubbery and sandstone-colored homes below his feet.

WHEN THE 13TH of January had finally arrived, my mother remembers walking to the doors of the university hospital, shivering not only from anxiety, but from the cold morning air. And then without pause, she remembers the waiting room at Washington University on that blistery morning. She had been waiting since September—been waiting for this renowned neurologist, Dr. Holtzman, to unlock a mystery inside her husband, who at the time sat calmly that morning by her side if not relaxed then sluggish. When my mother is nervous she becomes agitated. She tries to read magazines but focuses more on the length of time that passes, trying to manage her nerves before they choke her, restricting her breathing in the form of an asthma attack. Her breaths often squeak like the floors in our home early in the morning in her bedroom, when she would awaken and make her way down into the basement. Since September, she had been researching both on the Internet and in the public library—she had been researching *dementia* and what exactly that entailed for my father and his mind. And shortly after that first diagnosis he received in December of 1998, she discovered the symptoms and the signs of a disease named Pick's disease. And it was that disease that she had believed might be the cause of all of the mysteries. Pick's disease, unlike Alzheimer's, usually affects the younger age bracket, affecting personality before anything else, then speech impairment, and a reduction of coordination ability until the sufferer becomes akin to any other patient with dementia—immobile and mute. It wasn't completely gratifying to know that her husband might be suffering from it, but at least she had a name for what it was that was stealing him away from her. She had been at Washington University just a year before, right after the original neurologist had suspected dementia. Yet, the second prognosis was depression. Would she finally know a truth of some sort? Some sort of answer?

In the waiting room she sat with my father and the last few months of her silent, stressful research played out inside her mind until my father's name was called and they were led into Dr. Holtzman's office. I wish I could have known they were at the hospital that day—I wish someone would have told me what exactly was going on during those months my father stopped working and so seemed most happy and at ease, while my mother was just the opposite. I fought bitterly with her during those months, hitting her when she would raise her hands to me, pulling me off the ground by my hair and wildly hitting my back as she yelled to God for strength. I wish I could have known because maybe I would have been different. Maybe I would have sat in class instead of skipping most days, leaving in my Volvo station wagon to find a quiet spot to cry and chain smoke out the window—trying to appease a sickness I felt that had neither name nor cause. I'd sit with my arm dangling out the window, the smoke dancing above my wrist and into my eyes, and tears would form both from myself and the heat, and I never stopped to imagine my mother staring helplessly into Dr. Holtzman's eyes that morning. Her own tears she would know to stifle— even in her most trying times, she always seemed much stronger than me.

He started with tests, another MRI, again, questions from the past used to pinpoint changes and create a timeline of change. My father answered willingly and calmly, even happily. Since he stopped working, his entire demeanor had changed. He was docile and easily entertained. And most importantly, he was unaware. Of anything. Though he tried to pretend that he wasn't.

It was the moment she had wanted most since September, and it was finally here. She would finally know—and she trusted Dr. Holtzman. More than she trusted the others. Yet, "dementia" again was the prognosis—"I suspect Pick's disease" the latest addition.

My mother was numb. It was like watching the past few months again on repeat without sound. And in those moments she'd sit before the books in the library, the bright screen in the basement, the only words she'd see were "Pick's disease," "Alzheimer's disease"—was "dementia." She'd kept seeing that screen, and each time the desire to be wrong overtook her. But she wasn't wrong. She had been right all along.

She left right away—got up to leave the stifling air in Dr. Holtzman's office. She was upset, thinking to herself how much she wanted to be wrong, how much she wanted him to have depression. Simply just depression like the others had said. Maybe a little higher dosage of medicine, a little less of one in exchange for another. Surely that could be all. Surely that was it.

It may have started snowing, or the air may have sharpened the instant she left the office and began to cry. She stood by the window in the waiting room she and my father had sat in moments before. I wonder if she felt the cold through the windowpane as the secretary gently approached her. She led my mother to the research department where a year before she and my father had been interviewed, taped and sent away with only a syndrome marked in his file, "severe depression" scrawled in black. This day, she led my mother to speak with a researcher, to make my father a part of their research—the youngest man to be studied in the Alzheimer's Research Department at Washington University.

"A syndrome—why would they say that? The way they said it—it just did not sound as bad" were her thoughts a year later as she sat inside the research center. But the nurse sat beside her as my mother used her shoulder for a hug, and outside, sitting gleefully beside himself and staring at nothing really but the cookie he ate, my father felt content.

As I MADE room for my CDs, made space for my necklaces, my rings, and my bracelets, my father was outside somewhere or inside wandering around our summer home. More specifically, really, he was somewhere in his mind where none of us could read him except for the wisp of a sigh, falling on the ground behind his slow steps. And my mother who again began another running list in her mind of whether or not she needed the town's illusion of strength to hold her up. She still did not know if she should move us there or if the town had given her all the strength it possibly could. Only she could decide—and she was growing more confused by the day.

Unlike past summers when my parents spent the evenings walking around the town with friends and family, that summer they became fixtures at Franca's restaurant in the Piazza del Popolo. Franca's daughter Claudia and I became close friends. She saw in me in an instant something similar—a similar unhappiness, a stunted sense of complacency. I spent the summer alongside my cousin Claudio as well, finding in him a friend and a relative, feeling not quite so alone in my Pacentro self.

The first time I met with Claudio that summer in his kitchen, Zio Marco had already finished dinner. Claudio looked at me, almost smirking, and seemed to study my dress, my way of looking downwards. After my parents settled farther into their seats, commencing to stories, and my father sat chuckling, not really adding much to the conversations that surrounded him, Claudio motioned for me to stand up.

"Vieni—ti faccio conoscere qualcuna," he said to me as we walked downstairs, heading towards the door. I was interested to know whom he had in mind for me to meet. I felt an immense sense of elation come over me as I thought about how he thought he knew me already, knew me enough to have me follow him out the door leaving my family upstairs.

And then I met Claudia. She sat among a group of boys with her black hair cascading over her shoulders in spirals of curls, and she smiled.

Claudio led me and Claudia down past the Piazza Iaringhi, leading us past the ledge where people often rest to sit admiring the daylight or revel in the dark. We walked on past elderly couples walking arm in arm—or braccio sotto braccio, as I would come to learn. I would be part of that walking style soon enough with Claudia on my arm, giggling and concocting plans to escape from the town.

Finally, Claudio led us behind the ledge, beside an old house made of the same stone on which we were walking and the steps on which we were descending. And as Claudio doled out cigarettes to me and Claudia, we three sat and reintroduced ourselves through stories while I mainly listened and stumbled in Italian. I understood for the most part what was asked and what was spoken between the two, but for me speaking was still difficult. Perhaps not in the same way as my father, who was probably still sitting beside my mother with his hands folded against his chest. I could imagine him still wearing that smile and echoing laughs when it was appropriate. Yes, my stutters were different. I wasn't forgetting. I was in the process of remembering.

"MA, CAN I go to the beach with them? Come on, Ma." I looked at her, softening my tone as I ignored asking my father. It was now definitely clear to me that the shift had already commenced. I no longer asked him for permission; I nearly ignored his presence altogether. He was like a light fixture in a sunlit room—his authority was useless unless my mother wasn't around. And even in those moments, it wasn't the same as it was before because I knew I was taking advantage of him.

She said yes and I left to spend that week drinking, laughing and growing closer to my cousin especially. I didn't think twice about wearing shorts and bathing suits with my scratches on my legs for the world to see.

"Era un gatto di mio amico—" I told them all that first day at the beach. I blamed it on a cat: the pink scars on my legs and the slashes on my arms. I seemed to think a language barrier and my choppy sort of explanation could keep it all hidden. It wasn't until that first night, after my cousin and his friends were asleep, that I told Claudia about what I was doing to myself. She tried to understand me as I searched for words in Italian to match the words I experienced at home—and somehow she did. Somehow, she knew just how to react to make my feelings justified. She hugged me, uttering phrases my mother used to use as I lay in bed as a child. Back when I would lie between her and my father, as they tried to calm me, to soothe me. They tried to get my coughing to stop just by showing me more affection. And Claudia, sharing the same language as my mother, reached me that night through the same words I heard so many years before.

IT HAD BEEN years since those nights when I kept them up with my coughing. The nights I had the two of them together and I was the only thought of each. The way they loved me out loud even when they didn't speak a word. The way my mother held my hand, moving her thumb around my fingers, caressing my arm as I lay beside her. The way my father would be the first to stick up for me even when I didn't always deserve it. The way he'd go jogging and come back home with a turtle—the way they looked at me when I misbehaved and the peace that kept our spirits high when I didn't.

This love seemed altogether gone with the wind that carried it away. The absence left a different version of ourselves in a home where all I knew was rage and an ostensible desire to go back to the past.

But if I were to think back on an exact cause for those moments of my nearly ritualistic patterns of sitting on my floor, my back against my bed, holding onto whatever tool I chose with my right hand—I don't believe one would surface. The reasons are mixed in with the past, with the future I couldn't seem to change. They are in the beads of blood that somehow escaped me—the blood like pearls; I'd often wear them proudly. That's how I felt at times when I could see just what I felt on my arm. It was a war-zone, a landscape surrounded by streams, eradicated before the blood would drip onto the carpet. At times I chose my legs, my feet. And I would lie down, feeling the pulsing sting and shame but also victory. I was making myself suffer his pain. I took the sounds from our home—my mother's screams from downstairs, "Giovanni! I can't take it anymore!" and his angry protests and their fights—I took the sounds I heard and wore them. Converting them to my own blood.

I could sense their fights changing. My mother screamed more and my father became more violent. He seemed to grab her more, shake her more, and stop. He'd hit his head against the wall. And my mother's patience was slimmer. She wore her anger on her tongue and it would whip our backs. Now I can see she did it to soothe the sores of her wounds while I would run the blade across my arm, while Nicole rode her bicycle with her friends, and Flavia lay on a beach chair in our backyard.

Back in 1996 the police took them both in after my mother called them. She had warned my father not to hit her. That day when Flavia and I came home we knew something was wrong. We listened to Linda's message and made our way into her whitewashed sanctuary. We sat away from our grandmother who walked unsteadily from room to room, suffering already from dementia. With Linda and her family, we felt safe. The love she and her family had for all of us was our constant, our unchanging love.

My father stopped working just months before Nicholas's first birthday. Linda had gotten into the habit of bringing him over when my mother was home with my father. They would talk, drink coffee and coo over Nicholas as he looked about with his large blue eyes. My father would sit in his green recliner—but instead of staring silently ahead, he'd play with Nicholas, playfully chasing him around the room with his voice like Donald Duck.

After the visits, my mother would clean up the coffee cups and the cookies and sit beside my father, who would most likely still be wearing the faint signs of the smiles he had worn before. It was during those calm moments that my parents' love began changing.

I wonder how many afternoons they spent together in that living room before my father looked at my mother with steady eyes and a calm and humble demeanor.

"Enida," he said to her, though I don't know how or where. I only know for sure that the words came out as clearly as they had once before. "I'm sorry I never loved you the way you deserved to be loved," he would have continued to say without hesitation. "I love you. And I am so lucky to have you."

I wonder how she told Linda what my father had told her, changing their own love into a constant, unrelenting love. Different from before, as though my father were taking my mother's hand in his to face the Pacentrano sun and the steep and shadowed cliff of the Maiella Mountain. Their love had returned to its beginnings and it was in between the worst of fights that he realized how truly in love with his wife he actually was.

CLAUDIA AND I spent nearly every day together that summer in 2000. We shared many moments together, reliving experiences that were exciting, and exciting because they were wrong. After I told her everything that night, her perception of me seemed to change. She saw in me someone she hadn't seen before: I think she confused me with strength.

Though she failed in understanding me, I did feel as though she was my gift that summer; she was what I needed. We stole wine from her mother's bar and would drink it down those same steps Claudio led us down that first night we met. We would sit and drink, smoke cigarettes and write lyrics to songs we loved on the stones that surrounded us. Claudio would later join us and we'd drive down the Monte Morrone and into the town of Sulmona. We were always going somewhere, avoiding the squares and the people in them. Yet I couldn't always seem to hide myself from the stares of my father and my mother, who would sit hour after hour, talking with Franca, Claudia's mother, and various other Pacentrani. I'd approach them only when I needed something or felt the urge for family, but that would quickly dissipate. I would see Nicole hanging on our parents' arms, trying to get my father's attention.

It had been a strange year for Nicole—one of realization, above all else. Just a few months before leaving, she had been face to face with the disease and finally saw its shadowy outline in my father's falterings. In her Pokémon tee shirt and shorts, she stood beside him in line for a Saturday Pokémon tournament at Toys "R" Us.

"He took me a couple times—well, usually I went with friends, I guess. But daddy took me that afternoon. That I remember, Stef," she tells me, looking out my bedroom window after I ask her when it was that she first noticed his changes.

They had to be registered at the tournament, and as the man with the clipboard looked at my father, he asked him, "Zip code please?" And my father cleared his throat.

Nicole tells me she didn't even know what a zip code was at that time—at nine years old, she had spurted out the area code, instead. When that failed, the man awkwardly let them in. And Nicole looked up at her father with a hint of pity and fear. But she swallowed it down, just like I had done, just like we all had—until finally, we couldn't possibly ignore it any longer.

So as Nicole let go of her father's arm that summer, she went along and played and ran with friends her own age, as I kept my distance, wanting just to be away and to be free. Of course, I thought being free meant being apart from my family. I'd catch them randomly around the town. They'd stop and look and tell me, "ciao," and I'd nod and keep walking on, though I always felt them—their eyes, I could sense them. And yet, when I'd sit with my legs hanging over the balcony's edge, I'd think about how truly closed everyone else's eyes seemed to be. It is strange how much we fail to observe. Oddly, as everyone else failed to notice him, my mother's attention become much more keen.

That summer was the first time she really *smelled* his forgetting. "Giovanni? Did you use soap?" she asked him, as he'd sit with us downstairs, at the table or on the sofa.

"Yes," he'd say with a nod, a look of astonishment. Though he may not have known at all that he was lying. I'm sure he imagined the right way to wash, imagined the right way to shave, though at both, he failed.

So my mom stepped in the bathroom those afternoons when he showered and would call to him to use the soap, wash his hair with shampoo and remind him to rinse before he got out.

I listened from the sofa downstairs as the slight wind brushed my face, holding my chin up in its breeze. The warmth floats across my skin as I remember her telling him how to bathe and how to shave—I let my body rise and drift along with the air that flows against me.

And even on the balcony, I'd hear her start to tell him, "Giovanni—come here," as she'd help him dress. It was all becoming as real as the rough cement I dragged my knuckles against beside me.

I knew that every step they took among those people they were fooling was heavy and full. They were heaving with a need for comfort that, in the end, they didn't find that summer. My mother finally came to know that this disease was to fall on her; the disease was to be her fight. I guess she may have known that months ago after she raised her head from sobbing in her hands. After gently closing her phone book, she'd have thrown the book gently in a drawer.

We only had each other. I heard it from every breath of movement in our house that summer, and in the wind that carried with it our future and our hope. My father stood close by my mother that summer in Pacentro in a way he never had. They stayed together that summer as one.

On an afternoon, as I was sitting shotgun beside my cousin Claudio, listening to Korn on the radio, tapping my foot against the floor of his car as we sped down the Monte Morrone on an afternoon spent drinking beer beneath the coniferous trees up the mountain, I spotted my father. He was standing with his hands clasped behind his back. He wore a polo shirt tucked into his jeans. I could see the crisp fold of his collar as we approached in the car. My father gazed out into the Valle Peligna as he stood by the curve before La Madonnina, who stood solemn, her hands held up towards the sky.

And in a moment, my father turned his head. We looked at one another through the windshield, keeping each other's gaze just long enough for me to coolly turn away.

Chapter 8

Flavia had come to Pacentro in July to spend a few weeks with us before we returned home. I dreaded her visit. I knew that somehow she'd find a way to change it—that somehow, she'd find a way to spoil the little refuge I had built. Sitting in the backseat of Claudio's car, using makeshift ashtrays in the back as I chain-smoked along with Claudia and others, we'd listen to any music that might crack the foundations of the old homes and turn the crippling elder eyes that entombed us.

"I feel like you're crowding me—you're watching me *all* the time!" I would scream at her.

"Stef—maybe you *need* to be watched! Goddamnit! You are only sixteen!" Flavia would yell back.

"She's right, Stefa. I don't know who you think you are," my mother would begin, until her voice would rise higher and higher into a scream and I would escape to the balcony, and sit against the stone column. I would sit there for hours, until the sun would shift in the sky and the light from the day blended into evening. Then, I'd smell the scents of dinner coming from the kitchen and soon hear my mother's cries to come set up the table.

It was the last night we were in Pacentro in 2000, and my friends were waiting on me to join them at dinner. There they sat at a table among many, their laughter bouncing along the ridges in the walls behind them, and in the crevices of the leaves of the garnishing plants. They were eating pizza—Claudio, Claudia, and a few others, Michele, Maria Laura, Gabriella—the ones I'd spent the summer with and grew close to. The ones I felt betrayed by when Flavia made her presence known a few weeks before when she had come to visit us as well.

She was twenty and older than all of them. Claudio, who was eighteen at the time, felt like he knew her, and in my eyes, bonded with her differently. Now I can see how right he was to trust her more than me. She could have fun with them—speak more fluently than me, smile more than me. Flavia was serious when she needed to be, most often when dealing with me. But she could also laugh, could make jokes, could go far with her humor that seemed to supersede any fumbles or mistakes she made.

But that night, Flavia approached me as I stood among my friends besides Franca's bar in the Piazza del Popolo.

"Stef, I need to talk to you," she stammered as her reddened face grew colder and the little red circular mark beneath her right eye, the one that only seems to show when she's crying, stared at me equally as painfully.

"No, get away from me—" I said, pushing her away with my indifference as I tried to ignore what she just said.

"Now, Stef. I swear to god—" she started.

"Shut the fuck up, Fla. I'm not. This is my last night. I'm staying here," I said, more angrily than I can now reasonably justify.

"I read your diary—"she started.

And I lost my breath.

FLAVIA HAD SPENT the majority of that summer between her college in Illinois and our home in Chesterfield. That was the summer after her sophomore year in college. Since Flavia had left for college the year before, Nicole had kept a picture of Flavia on her bedroom wall—an eight-and-a-half by eleven portrait, and it hung between the two windows in her pink bedroom. The sadness she kept for Flavia's absence was as real as the hopelessness I felt at the time. Her sophomore year, Flavia had started seeing a psychologist. And she says with complete conviction—"I went mainly because of you. And then for dad." Somehow, I didn't realize that I truly was becoming more fatal than my own father's illness.

During her time alone at home that June, Flavia had decided to do what she could to change me. So one afternoon, she stepped into my room with a bucket of paint and a brush and started to paint my bedroom walls white. Perhaps the exact moment I was outside in Pacentro, on my balcony or out with Claudia, Flavia threw sheets on my furniture and laid paper upon the floor. And as she dipped her brush and ran it smoothly across the walls, she suddenly noticed how far I had gone. It was a surprise she later told me—a surprise in the worst sense to see the markings I had made, the phrases I had written during my rituals of harm, the blood that dried after I'd wipe my arms against them. She painted through her shock and pushed herself through the moments where she'd have to breathe and wonder how I could have possibly done this to myself, least of all to them.

I know she must have wanted to stop. I would have. But she didn't. She stood firmly and defiantly because it wasn't in her to stop. She pushed through whatever dread she may have felt and replaced it with determination to rid myself of myself by somehow cleaning away my past before I had a chance to return to it.

Her voice I couldn't hear as she told my mother over the phone that she had painted my room. Replacing my things that I had accumulated, my meaningless things that I had acquired, with my old china dolls I had once collected. The dolls were dusty, I'm sure of it, as she struggled to reach for them up into my closet. The sun emanating inside my room from outside my window perhaps made the endeavor that much more exhausting. And as her glistening body, wet from the sweat of trying to change what she could not, sat for a moment to see the room she had recreated, I wonder if she felt content. I seem to think more and more that maybe she lies when she tells me I think too much of the past. I seem now to believe she holds more hope and nostalgia than I could ever have thought possible.

But when Flavia read my diary that night she approached me and demanded I speak to her about what I had written, I didn't find her nostalgia at all admirable. We walked into a small side road away from the piazza. The ground was white from the stone that glowed beneath the moonlight and the homes on either side of us seemed vacant.

We discussed the contents of the diary and I told her I would never trust her again. I told her I hated her. I told her I felt raped. She had read my thoughts that I was not willing and ready to share. They were temporary, I had believed. They were mine. Yet, she had read them. Read the words over and again at times. And maybe the hardest part for her through all of it was realizing that my newly painted walls might as well have been left the same after all.

ON THE PLANE ride back to America I had no idea what Flavia had done to my bedroom until that night when I opened the door and stepped in. I gathered up all the dolls once more and hid them away in my closet. I returned to my life at home as though nothing were altered but the thickening anger I held for Flavia and most everyone else for that matter. All that I seemed to hold dear was the idea that I had left behind my true friends back in Italy. I had left behind two months of escape and happiness. I had spent two months pretending I could be fine on my own.

THE SEPTEMBER AFTER our trip, I started my junior year in high school and Flavia left for her junior year in college. Nicole entered the sixth grade and my father became incontinent.

I was in the kitchen putting dishes away when I heard the garage door open. My mother entered and walked quickly upstairs. I paid little attention to my father until I noticed he had remained standing where my mother had left him. He was standing quietly beside the garage door with tears rolling down his cheeks. It was the first time he had had an accident, soiling himself during a walk with my mother. His gray sweatpants were soaked and darkened and his back was bent forwards in shame. I don't remember telling him not to worry. I don't remember telling him it would be all right—that I loved him just the same.

Instead, I took the moment like I did the others, and stashed it away inside my mind to relive again and again when I'd sit inside my room. Or, I'd reveal them in moments of frustration when I would talk to my best friend, Dan, on his rooftop.

Dan and I became friends when we were just beginning to be teenagers. We met in middle school when we were twelve. I began to dress in black and he began to join groups made exclusively of women. I remember the day we became friends. He was sitting in the hallway with three other girls. They had just made a name for their group—JadS—an acronym from each of their names. I remember rolling my eyes at the thought upon first hearing and later sitting down in science class. We were assigned to sit beside each other in the back corner of the classroom at a large table. It may have been the best moment I spent in class. It was to be the day I'd meet my best friend.

"Today's the anniversary of my dog dying," he told me as he flipped through his large three-ring binder that took up most of the room on our table. Dan has a look in his eyes when he's about to take the conversation down a strange and wonderful path. It's above a look of sarcasm, more than a challenging look or a look of feigned innocence. There's something intelligent in the way his eyes sparkle and entice you further. At the time, his hair was cut into a bowl haircut and he wore tee shirts and collared shirts and sneakers most days. His eyes are hazel though they often shine through green. "Daisy," he continued, "died a few weeks ago. The Kennel she was staying at killed her when my family and I were in Hawaii," he told me matter-of-factly. I even noticed a smirk—he knew he was making me uncomfortable and that's what he was hoping for.

"Oh—" I started, not really knowing what to say but thinking he was strange for telling me. And in such a strange way, he was mourning her with me.

Shortly afterwards, we got yelled at by our teacher for talking and laughing in class. Apparently, my introduction to Dan through his dead dog was all we needed to break the ice.

Dan and I quickly became fused together in every sense of the words of trouble, of fun. In middle school, we'd crawl out his window and walk atop his roof and watch the cars drive by his home. He'd offer me coffee from his coffee pot he kept beside his fish tank when we were only starting high school. And junior year, when my family was really beginning to change, Dan was waiting for me amid the sounds of his jungle animal wall clock, each hour chiming to the tune of a lion or a parrot. By that time, Dan had already started coming out to his specific friends one by one, to me by way of a poem he had written—"you're sterile?" were my first words I asked him as I sat on his counter in his kitchen. He had just concluded his lines with a fear he keeps inside—of never having kids of his own, a family to call his own. At sixteen, we were still too young to understand the road that would lead to Dan's realization that one day, he *would* be able to imagine at least the possibility, though that afternoon, with my legs swinging against the cupboards, I still felt the urge to play along with Dan that his secret was safe with me.

And my secrets, too, were safe with Dan. "He shifts the gear—he'll put it in neutral, in Drive 1 or 2 just randomly—and he drives an automatic," I would tell Dan, as we'd sit on his roof. Invariably, I would be smoking a cigarette during our talks, amid Dan's objections that they were making his contacts dry out and his migraine flair up. He would have me pay him three dollars a cigarette each morning he drove me to school—and still, I'd ignore his complaints, his attempts at making me stop.

Dan never really knew what to say those times I let my guard down. I was angry in those instances and it was suffocating me, changing *me* and turning me into someone I never thought possible.

The anger ran through me and the only way I knew how to appease it was through cutting, through smoking, through drinking, through fighting with my mother and going inside myself more and more until I thought I could blame my actions solely on my invisible demons—my depression, my confidant, my friend.

Yet, Dan had ways to reach me in the moments I needed him. And it's clear to me now, thinking back to those nights on his rooftop when I would just cry and he would just listen and then we would go back inside. It's clear to me now that all I needed was to be heard because I needed to say the words out loud—my father was sick, my father was sick, my father was sick—and perhaps this mantra would finally make the words sound familiar and ultimately so meaningless that it would bring me back to the girl I had left behind.

Thinking back now, I wonder why I didn't use Dan's friendship more positively. Instead, he was another form of keeping a diary, a way to write down my secrets and the thoughts I kept hidden from those around me. Like the cuts I kept hidden, so I kept my secrets encased in my hackneyed version of strength that I assumed was impenetrable. But if my father was teaching me anything at that moment, it was the realization that I was just as weak as my defenses were. My ways of coping were just as useless as my anger was.

For on one afternoon, I found myself sitting on my bed and slashing meekly, then more deeply. Just a few here and there mainly where a watch could hide it or a ribbon. I often saved the lasting scars for when the nights were extra dark, during a shower in the day, any moment really when I found my breathing scarce and stifled. On this particular day, I found myself simply cutting to recharge myself, making myself ready and willing to lie beside my mother on the couch and pass the time watching television.

Afterwards, I walked into the living room with my wrists adorned in shoelaces and a watch, hair ties and a lace.

"Stefa—why are you wearing all those bracelets?" My mother asked me as she looked at me from where she lay on the couch.

"I don't know," I told her, hoping it would silence her. I lay down on the couch beside her, after just sitting in my room the past few hours. I had been reading a book, trying to see if I could find some meaning in a word or two, and suddenly sadness overtook me, and anger and anxiety and a feeling that it could all lessen if I were to just open up my closet door, reach beneath my junk box on the second shelf, and pull out my red Swiss Army knife with General Electric written in white on the side. I had taken it from my father's desk drawer one afternoon while rifling through his things.

At one point, I got up from the couch and went back to my room. I left my mother lying there and the phone rang and I didn't move. It was Flavia—"Mom, I'm worried about Stef. It's not normal how she acts—and I think she might be hurting herself—" I could imagine her starting, and my mother, her initial reaction was to hunt for the truth, bitterly, with fear.

"Stefa! Vieni qua!! Come downstairs, NOW! Sbrigati!" She screamed from the bottom of the steps. I imagined she was mad about a cigarette she found beside the bush against our house again. Maybe I left the kitchen a mess like I had already done before. Maybe I did something, anything, but it surely wasn't what I had thought that afternoon I walked calmly down the stairs as my mother snatched my wrists in her hands and screamed.

A few hours later, after my room had been torn to pieces and my hair lay like torn weeds across the floor, after Nicole sat beside me crying and my mother examined my body—"You said these were blisters you shaved over—Naggia Cristo!" She'd yell after finding other markings and the moment my father walked into my room, repeating the words, "Unbelievable" over and again. I didn't think I could feel more evil, more wicked, than the moment I had to hand him my knife, and my father fell down and wept.

Of course, my mother did the same for me, quickly replacing her anger with patience as she lay with me that night after I lay on my bed, picking at my arms in desperation, trying to find a layer to hide myself within.

I HAD TO attend outpatient therapy at a hospital for a week. It was about twenty miles from our home. That first day, my dad, neatly showered and shaved with the help of my mother, had driven me. He was still driving at this point, though less than he used to. It would be several months before Flavia would tell my mother how scared she felt driving with him in the car and my mother would finally make the decision that would reverberate with a sense of finality I hadn't yet felt.

"Stefania, I love you, you know that?" He told me, and I breathed a sigh as tears fell from my eyes and I hugged him. I held him for a second longer than I normally would have and walked beside him to the building that would hopefully try and fix me.

The building was an extension of the hospital that stood behind it. When I walked in beside my father, I noticed the waiting room had pamphlets showcasing young teenagers smiling with words of hope splayed out above them. Other pamphlets simply had young people sitting in the fetal position, hiding, it seemed, from the sadness that we shared. I grew annoyed at these pamphlets and these papers that promised to understand me, heal me—perhaps even change me. What did I need to change for? I wasn't sick. My father was.

As he guided me through the hallways, he walked strongly. I remember I did feel safer beside him. And I don't recall him speaking to anyone in particular. We just roamed the halls, searching for a room number.

We finally did find it and when we opened the door, we were met with another hallway of doors on one side, and on the other, a solemn doorway that stood open. Inside, I spotted people my own age, sitting in chairs, talking with one another; I even heard some laughing.

But we kept walking straight, straight into the room that was the largest and had, on one side, an office with glass on all sides. There, several nurses were writing notes, organizing files, and looking up one by one.

All of the specifics of this building are simple paint strokes on a canvas that seems unsteady. I can barely make out any of these specifics because they're dim, dreary, and hazy. If I try too hard to remember it all, my memory fades completely and I am left with just the inkling of a vision of my father stepping away. He becomes the walls I can no longer see in that room at the outpatient hospital. His eyes glide along the edges of the floor around his feet. And I am left calling out his name, yelling for him to come back to me, come get me. As the nurses take my blood pressure and write notes down in my file, I turn my head to find him and he is gone.

I WAS SENT to go sit in that room where the others were. It was a room filled with chairs on either side, a small couch against a wall and a table in the center. I sat on the safest chair I could find—it was next to the door and separated from everyone else. They looked at me and tried to study me until one of them asked me, "Why you here? What's wrong with *you*?" As though I were joining a club of fellow troubled teens that somehow wanted to rate me based on my form of neurosis.

"I cut myself," I told them all. Emotionlessly, I looked at their uncaring faces and then I stared at the ground and waited for the day to finally be over.

The room I was in grew more and more stifling as I sat there, feeling judged by these people who likely felt just as anxious as I did. At one point, I got up and went to the nurses' station. I stood motionless, my body taut, as I stared into a television screen with nothing but the room I was in, and the faces and the words of all of my fellow patients. There was a nurse who seemed specifically assigned to watch us and take notes of our behavior. I felt a surge of panic run through me. Again, it seemed I couldn't escape. I couldn't find anything that was truly mine.

A few days later a nurse took my blood pressure as she did each day. But that morning I had worn a jacket to cover my cuts on my arm, the frantic scabs from pinching my arm while my mother stood before me screaming. I had done something, I don't remember what, but it had upset her and I had felt angry. Angry enough to push myself again to hurt myself. The nurse forced me to take my jacket off and when she saw my arm, she sent for my parents.

I sat on the couch waiting for each of my parents to come in and hear the news that I hadn't stopped. I would never stop, at least for several years after that afternoon.

"I swear—I swear I'll get better. I won't do this again. I promise," I said to them that day as I sat between them both following the meeting we had with a nurse. And it was the first time I sat between them that I knowingly lied about never again hurting them both purposefully. I hid my face behind my long hair that sprawled against my lap. Just an hour before, my father had received the phone call from the nurse and arrived before my mother. Tearing his jacket off he asked exasperatingly, "What happened? What's the matter?" He couldn't have imagined that I would do it again.

"I will stop. I will get better. I'm sorry," I choked until finally, somehow, they believed me. And I went back to learning how to cope with my emotions, to learning how to fix my own illness that lay suffocating my family in vain. And whether or not I succeeded didn't matter. All that really mattered was that I didn't give up.

But my father had dementia. That much I knew for certain. And I knew it every minute, and every time I lost control, making mistakes, smoking even marijuana on school grounds one afternoon the year before—weeks after having first tried it, I decided to take the chance, skip class and smoke on the grounds of my former middle school.

"Please—please don't tell my parents. My father—my father, don't. He's sick. He's sick and I can't do this to him," I pleaded with the principal I had known well just a few years before when I had first started wearing black and dangling ribbons on my wrists.

My attempts didn't prevail and I found myself, not too long afterwards, sitting across from members of the school board, my principals from high school. They would suspend me for two weeks, but before my sentencing I was to explain myself. And while I sat between my mother and my father, each of us cried, it seemed, for just the same reasons.

I didn't want to keep hurting them—I surely didn't want to keep hurting my father, who in the past year had cried more times than I had ever known him to before. I was chipping away at all he had left and it was just a matter of time before I would crush him entirely, if the dementia didn't do it first. And it was all I could do to not end it all before that fear would become a reality.

PART III

Summer 2000 – Summer 2002

Chapter 9

My mother always walks ahead of us. She seems to think she is always rushed—even when it's obvious she isn't. But her mind works that way. Its movement keeps her steady; its grit gives her strength. I believe her frantic desire to move forward in haste is what made my mother's journey to bury her husband that afternoon possible.

I must have been clearly out of sight from her. I must have walked paces slower than my mother. Nicole, though she complained, kept steady with my mother. She knew it was not a time to start a fight. I did as well, but I am prone to laziness and because of that, I often find myself at the center of an argument. But at that time, I tried to forgo my own penchant for second guessing my mother's rush. I can still feel the pull towards my mother, towards my uncle who I knew was waiting for us at the arrivals gate.

I don't remember it clearly, the afternoon we walked through the paths and halls, through the people and the language that must have felt soothing and welcoming. The Italian they spoke, hurried, like my mother's footsteps, reminded me of home and of my father. The idea of returning was settling upon me day after day and it must have felt, in a way, nearer to completion as I followed my mother. Following my mother, I felt safe.

Walking through the vanishing shades of light, I imagine us passing through customs, gathering ourselves together before entering the crowded doorway of the arrivals gate. I see my mother pass through before me, before my sister, and from the sides of her I can spot faces smiling and calling out to those around us. I can feel the anxiety catch within my throat and my eyes fall on the blue luggage my mother dragged behind her. And I feel at long last the expectant moment of our arrival, of the years behind me melting into these specific moments. I see my uncle, Zio Marco, standing beside himself, one arm bent at his side, his palm against his hip. Near him, I see Flavia searching earnestly for our eyes among the crowd.

"Ciao Marco—" my mom started, as she fell inside his open arms. I heard her gasps between her cries as I looked at them both. It was different this arrival. It was different in the way he held her, and it surely was not the embrace I had expected from him. In the ways I was my sisters' sister, he was again, my mother's brother.

I grasped on to Flavia as hard as I could, knowing she gets uncomfortable when I do. And as my mother let go of her brother, I fell into him as my mother had and held onto him a little bit longer than I would have. We stood, the five of us, beside our luggage. I felt the warmth from the sun I could see from the windows surrounding us. I could feel the fear in me that day, as I knew the burial approached us even closer—but I also felt the bond that kept us there, separate from anyone else in the room. Our family stood for a brief moment and it was something else entirely different from the years we had come to that point before.

Finally, my uncle turned us around and we walked almost in single file through the doors that swished open automatically. Nicole decided to drive along with Flavia to Pacentro, leaving me alone with my mother and uncle. The sun was shining as I squinted after them, turning back around to face my mother. And she squinted just the same as she would after hours of staring into the computer screen in the basement of our home back in 2000, when she began reading websites devoted to caregiving and dementia.

AFTER WE RETURNED that summer in 2000, and I made my way up the stairs and into my newly redecorated room, I settled into a space that lay somewhere between my then-present self and my childhood. I yelled at Flavia as loud as I possibly could before slamming my door and forcing myself to sleep. It always takes a bit of time to readjust to my American Missouri self upon returning from Pacentro. And seeing my room as it was didn't make the transition any easier.

Downstairs, my sisters and my mother must have taken out the luggage, bringing them upstairs, before settling into their former selves again. And my father, I wonder what it must have felt like to not be able to really settle anywhere whatsoever. From my perch upon my bed, I imagined he must have sat down quietly into that green recliner, reached for the remote control and watched television. He knew to pick up right where he had left off. His actions were like reactions; movements made from stimuli, thoughtlessly carried out, like blinking.

And so, we came to live once more in our home after a summer spent away. But my mother still had not decided where she wanted to remain: in Missouri or Pacentro. "I don't—I don't know," she would whisper while she lay on her bed, her right arm draped over her eyes, her other clenching and releasing beside her. She would tell me Pacentro one week—"Stefa, yes. We are going to move there. I have no one here—no one cares. At least there I have family; I have my sisters. Yes, we'll move to Pacentro." And then the week would fall into another week—"Stefa, let's stay here. We have no one there. At least here, we will have a better life. There is nothing there."

And I went back to school as I had done, back to junior year, to working again at the movie theatre. And they would come at times together, getting their free popcorn, their free sodas, getting excited by the deals. My parents continued to live as partners, my mother keeping him busy, having a different form of marriage where the two became inseparable throughout the day. As I'd watch them enter into the theatres from where I stood behind the concession stand, I thought that must be bliss for them. Bittersweet for my mother—a fantastical monetary arrangement for my father.

But when I came home in the evenings, bypassing Nicole's school-work questions, my mother would be in the basement as before. Reading and rereading the screen, searching for anything that would help her help us. Every so often, she'd print off a copy of the caregiving discussion board to show Flavia or me, or she would reread the papers later by herself. A few times my mother called for me to come down and sit with her as she read the threads, even telling me to come over and read over her shoulder, trying to get me to see and understand what she had. But it never seemed to settle—that's the only explanation I can really seem to accept. How else could I continue to wake up, go to school and come home, without trying my damnedest to spend his last coherent months trying to *know* him—digging into my father's brain for pieces of him that I could collect, protect and keep with me throughout my life?

There was that one year when I was in sixth grade—the only time I had ever given my father an interview. About his life, I asked him questions—how it felt to leave Italy, live in Venezuela for a time—and finally, how it was that he got his blood mixed in with the cream he used to fill donuts in college. I sat in his office in the basement, while he shuffled around papers and took breaks with me, leaning back in his mustard yellow chair, laughing with me about a memory he shared. I scribbled down answers as fast I could and read them back to him, making sure I caught every nuance, every joke—every slight indication that it was my father who spoke and I who wrote.

I included photos of him throughout the years of his growing up. On the cover of the binder I bound it in, I put a large picture of the Italian flag with a title that has since disintegrated from my mind along with many of the details of that interview.

I would say it was about a year before I threw the pages out with the trash, heedlessly erasing that afternoon I sat with him in the basement. I had thrown away his jokes, the pauses where he'd stop to clear his throat—and an image of a man Nicole would never seem to remember.

MY UNCLE LED my mom and me to his car. It was one of the first times I can remember that he didn't come prepared with a van shaped like a large rectangular box. The vans in Italy have such a misshapen body compared to what we're used to in America. But I guess they just need them that way—easier when racing down two-lane highways cutting through caves and over tight bridges atop steep valleys. We didn't stall in the parking lot for long before Zio Marco found his way out and onto the busy highway. I don't remember clearly if he kept the radio on, though if he had, I'm sure I didn't hear much of anything besides the loud whir of the engine in his sedan as he sped, chain-smoking out the window.

I seem to wonder about the many times I have driven through Pacentro in the small, cramped car of my uncle, of my cousin Claudio—and notice the way they stare ahead—thinking of seemingly nothing at all. Reflecting on the times when I sat as a passenger, I often find myself contemplating the austere indifference of the town and the way it seems to echo through its people. Above the silence and the stress that comes from it, I manage to see my uncle as mimicking this beauty, driving silently, seemingly brooding. When I think of myself, of my sisters, I have the sense that we are still just actively inhaling the sights around us. My uncle, instead, seems to match the trees in his silent dismissal of their beauty. Even the way my uncle sits, hunched and slouching in his seat, seems to speak of another form of splendor I couldn't seem to imagine at home. And my mother, inside herself, maybe remembering, shares that image of belonging inside those mountains that run in waves outside her window of the car.

I wonder if my father had that same look in his eyes. I never thought to look. Or if I had, I don't remember. It seems strange what we do remember and what we don't. I remember my father taking me down the mountain to the town of Sulmona one afternoon in 2000 after my mother had refused to leave the couch. I remember the struggle he had parking and the fear I had in my throat, close to tearing, as we wound down the mountain. I remember how my father looked sitting in the chairs at Franca's bar in the Piazza del

Popolo with the sun behind him, shining on his bald spot. But I cannot see if the look in his eyes resembled the look of Zio Marco's—I rather assume it was different. Connected as he was to Pacentro, as my mother was to the town, my parents were temporary. Yet they did seem to gather strength from returning. They seemed to renew themselves by stepping back inside their lives that were left behind. Instead of growing used to the breeze that came from way up high in the Maiella Mountain range, their souls were rejuvenated by the air that enriched their blood with the gust of a thousand breezes.

WHAT MY MOTHER used to read on those threads were tales of horror—loved ones explaining away the day in order to make room for a second wind. They'd turn away slowly from the computer and return to the ones they love with mangled minds and have nothing but the satisfaction that maybe somewhere, maybe someone, knows exactly what they are saying when they write, "I'm tired. I feel like giving up. But I can't."

My mom never wrote, and I try to understand why she just wouldn't say even one thing—ask just one question—instead of looking in on a group of people who seemed to form a clique in their grief. Had my mother written in 2000, after we returned from Pacentro, she would have told them all how she was beginning to see the effects of my father's dementia much stronger than before. If her fears were a waterfall she imagined from the window of Dr. Holtzman's office, her hair would lay matted now above her slackened shoulders, and the window would now be shattered. Reading entry after entry on the Pick's disease caregiving websites or the Alzheimer's caregiving sites, she compared and contrasted her husband and envisioned him hanging from atop that surge of water where change only pushed him backwards and down within that gulf.

For in October, my mother was regularly showering my dad, shaving him, dressing him, brushing his teeth. At times, I'd look at him as he sat in front of the television in his green recliner and notice the precision with which my mother trimmed his mustache and his sideburns. "I don't understand men today—why they cut their sideburns so short. Back in the 70's we *wanted* them long—we fought for them to be long!" He told me once in the car as we drove up to a man who sat staring at the light, his sideburns nearly nonexistent. "See? Look at mine—*mine* aren't even that short!" He said. And I nodded in agreement, deciding right then and there to never respect a man who didn't respect long sideburns.

My mother seemed to know or at least remember that rule of my dad's regarding sideburns. She shaped them strongly, leveled and positioned confidently on his head—the gray in his hair adding even more prestige. He would smell strongly of aftershave, of Polo, most likely. And my mother would even dress him in a collared polo shirt even if he spent the day in his chair.

In the beginning, it was hard for me to imagine her showering him in their bathroom. I didn't understand if she went inside with him or stood outside with a washcloth or even just directed him on what to do next. When I would help Nicole shower, I would mainly tell her what to do and begrudgingly rinse the shampoo from her hair. I would try not to get too wet or, even worse, get my socks wet—I hated pulling off wet socks. But my mom—I wondered how she managed. How she sat him down after she dried him. How she made him face her as she delicately rubbed shaving cream on him, shaving him so expertly—he would hardly have a notion of a nick.

I see them through the opposite side of the mirror where I sense her strain. Her eyes fall at the edges; her mouth frowns. And he looks up at her just as she pauses. Her eyes drift towards a reflection of a wife and mother and back again at him. He waits for her gentle touch to hold his face in her hands once more. I catch the meaning of love and I realize this is it.

Chapter 10

Now that my father began sliding downwards ever faster, I started experiencing things at home differently as well. Perhaps it was a sense of loneliness I tried to stave off—though, if it were, my father would have been the forerunner in the attempt. Both he and I shared moments where our seclusion came spilling forth from ourselves—uncontrolled and unabated. My father had a better way of handling his isolation than me—as a well man, he knew how to keep his weaknesses away from me. Perhaps not true in my mother's estimation, but for me, he was the man who would travel always alone, calling me from whatever time zone he may have found himself in.

Normally, it would be through a phone call I'd answer absentmindedly that would remind me that he was indeed alone— "Hey, what are you doing?"

"Watching TV. Where are you?" I told him, as I slid down from the sofa and onto the floor.

"I'm in a Chinese restaurant," he said. And I knew he was waiting for my jealousy to erupt in a squeal—"You are!? I wish I was there!" As a child, I worshipped Chinese food. Back in Erie, Pennsylvania, I had locked myself by accident in the bathroom right before we were to leave for our favorite Chinese restaurant. I started pounding the door, crying and screaming. My parents pretended they would go without me—telling me I eat Chinese food too much anyway. Luckily though, I made it out that afternoon and managed to refrain from locking myself up again in that bathroom.

"I know. When I come home we'll go. OK?" And I assented. Though shortly afterwards, I felt a slight pang and asked him—"Dad?

Are you there by yourself?"

"Yes."

"Do you get lonely, daddy?" I asked him, feeling sad for him, wanting to be there with him.

"Yeah. I do—but it's OK, Stefania. I'm used to it." He sounded so sweet, I remember, so earnest. But he had called me during a moment when he sat alone at a restaurant. Most likely, thinking of us—I like to think he wished us there beside him. For some reason, him revealing to me that he was lonely made me feel even more connected to him. And a minute later, his food arrived and we said goodbye.

DURING MY SECOND semester of junior year in high school, Dan and I often traveled in his white Accord. I needed space, time to breathe away from my home, where my father and mother were like strewn pillows on the sofa, though still sitting in their respective places: my father on the recliner, my mother on the couch.

Dan knew just what I needed—just a bit of time with him alone, a few cigarettes and some coffee. On weekends, Dan would ask me, "Where do you want to go tonight?" But we'd already know the answer. "OK, but smoke out the window. My eyes are burning already."

We would go to a coffee shop called The Grind. It was in the city, not too far into the city, but just enough to make it about a twenty minute drive from our homes in the suburbs.

"Yeah, OK. But I gotta be back by 11:30," I told him, as I lit up a cigarette and blew the smoke out the window. "I just don't fucking understand though. I mean, I'm seventeen and I can't even go home past twelve. It's just fucking unbelievable!"

"Hey, it's OK—you have Italian parents . . . " Dan would say, smiling. "They're not from here."

"Shut up," I'd start. I'd feel the frustration grow inside me, feeling the need to cry but stifling it. Instead, I would turn up the music and we'd sing together; we'd laugh.

Dan, again, proved to be my salvation, my remedy, though often-times I preferred to be alone. Preferred perhaps is not the correct word—I *needed* time alone. That was how I dealt with it all—through the acts I'd do on my own. I'd let the feelings escalate and swell, like the waves of the ocean I used to love swimming in long ago.

Since my father got sick, I stopped loving going out as I had back then, back when I'd float to his side, rising and falling from the waves of his feet in front of me. I had tried to snorkel one day without him, during a family outing at the beach in Italy. But I soon found I couldn't get past the fear I had of all of the creatures beneath me, the fish surrounding me, the strange and foreign world below me. I remember stopping suddenly and finding sharp-nosed fish poking me in the feet, and I panicked. I almost drowned, swimming with all of my might to the shore. Throwing my snorkel gear in the sand, I picked up a book and started to read. I can't say when that day was exactly, only that it was the first of many times I realized that change was approaching me before I had a chance to acclimate myself to it.

DAN AND I entered The Grind and quickly became enveloped in smoky air that settled upon our skin. We stood in line and looked up at the white board, at all of the coffee drinks written in the familiar scroll and chose two house coffees—served in large white mugs. The woman at the register had shoulder-length black hair and thin eye-brows she drew on daily. She smiled at us and it seemed as though there was a chance she recognized us, though which one of us she recognized was anyone's guess. Dan and I had a running contest to see who would be recognized first through that question—"the regular?"

We took a seat at a round table somewhere among the others who we'd see week after week, some on laptops, others playing chess. And we'd begin our night with stories from the week or me beginning to open up about what it was that made me especially irritated that day.

"I can't stand her anymore, Dan. I feel like sometimes I want to kill her—" I'd start. "If not her, then myself."

My mother and me. Our relationship was growing ever-more tumultuous. When I'd come home in the night she was always awake. Waiting for me in the family room, waiting for me to approach her so she could smell my breath, checking for alcohol or cigarettes. Since the year before when I had been suspended for smoking marijuana on school grounds, any ounce of trust my mother might have had for me had vanished.

While I was out with Dan, she would always be home with my father. He would sit and stare at the television, perhaps look at my mother to try and say something, but get lost in his stutters and die away. They weren't getting along as they had before because now that his disease was settling comfortably within him, he seemed more angry, his mood swings more abundant. It was as though the disease was now stronger than him, and he knew it. Maybe he even let it be so. No doubt he was becoming depressed. And in that hazy existence, my father was seemingly giving up.

"They're fighting more too. Like before. I just can't take it. The other day she told me to clean. Clean. Clean! That's all she fucking says to me! She never talks, never does anything but go lie upstairs in her bed. So I screamed and threw the plates on the floor. She went up to me and started hitting me so I hit her back and called her a bitch or something I don't know—" I recounted.

"Stefania—she's just scared. Maybe that's all it is. I'm sorry—you just need to get out more," he said, taking a sip of his coffee from his hand that always seemed to shake. Dan was on so much medicine himself—antidepressants, medicine for his irritable bowel syndrome and vitamins I couldn't begin to name. My father, too, used to take vitamins. So many vitamins. So many, in fact, that I'd roll my eyes at him as he'd tell me, "Look Stefa—vitamins are good for you. You need to take them, Stefania. They'll make you stronger and make you live longer." I was then—and still am—an avid vitamin skeptic.

"Then when I slammed my door, she runs up and starts pounding it while I started scraping at my arm again. I cut the shit out of my arm—I wanted to kill myself," and at this, I start to cry remembering myself crouched behind my bed, digging my Swiss Army knife into my arm and jamming at it as though it were already dead. "Then I heard her calling Flavia again like she does *all* the time. Every fucking time!"

"Did she find out you cut yourself again?" He asked, looking worried. He knew about the last time when I had nearly destroyed my already weakening parents. He knew how I was punished, grounded, for harming myself and how much pain I would inevitably put my family through if they found out I had done it yet again.

"No—no she doesn't. Thank god it's cold outside, right?" I managed a smile as I took out another cigarette. I found great relief chain-smoking in that coffee shop—taking deep drags and exhaling as I looked around the walls, at the dark maroon and blue paintings, the dimly lit spaces between the patrons and the torn black leather couches—I felt at home there amid my synergistic surroundings.

MY MOM AND I didn't just fight about cleaning, about her nightly breath analysis or about my own vastly increasing mood shifts. A month before I started working at Wal-Mart that January, I walked up the stairs after my last day at the movie theatre and stood a moment in front of her open door where she lay. "Ma, I quit the movie theatre," then headed into my room and shut the door. I could hear her screaming and the recliner of my father's chair close, and soon, his steps on the stairs.

"Shut up!!" I screamed from my room.

"You better get another job! STRONZA!" She cried.

"Why? I'll find another fucking job!! Just shut the hell up!!" I could never take her screaming. It felt icy and jagged and it acted as the catalyst for my meltdowns. I didn't always try to upset her on purpose; never did I expect the reaction I received from her each time. But it always happened. Each and every time.

Though I hated her for telling me to get another job, I knew I needed to shut her up. I never was able to actually have my money I made. Instead, I'd sit in the backseat of my sister's car or my mother's car as they'd drive me to the bank and have it deposited. Any time I would make a withdrawal, one or the other would ask me why—what for—and doubt whatever answer I would give them. My father would tell me again and again it was for my own good in the little ways he could. "Stefania, you need to. Save. It's important," I can almost hear him tell me now. And I tried to follow his words, tried to make him see I knew the value of money. But I was still too young, too immature, too volatile to make them trust me. Perhaps they were correct in wanting to steer me directly. My mother made up for my father's mental absence through anger, however, and I didn't seem to learn much from her.

And Flavia made up for his absence through control. She seemed to take it upon herself to be the father in ways he never had with me. But their relationship was different—it had always been. Flavia and my dad fought more than I did with my dad when he was well—we were partners against them. And we found respite from them in the ways we bonded, in my feigned interest in the books he would read and recount to me, and in my eagerness to hide downstairs in the basement with him, playing foosball. "Dad—just one more game! One more!" But Flavia was four years older than me, and during her teenaged tempered years, she and my father often fought in front of me. So I didn't see them much the other way—the way she remembered. The way he would speak to her as a partner and as a father. The way he would give her advice for her future, eat with her at college on days he'd pass through on business. Instead, my father and I spent his best years as friends.

On our way to my interview at Wal-Mart, Flavia drove my father and me. "Stef, make sure you shake the manager's hand," she told me as we waited at a stoplight. He had wanted to join us—I see now he wanted to father me. He wanted to take part in the moment. "Stef—seriously, you have to shake his hand *firmly*."

And looking back, I see my father was nodding, agreeing with Flavia. He, too, shook my hand and tried to gauge the strength of it—the confidence of it. That's all they were seeking really, my confidence. But where I showed *them* little, I showed more than enough on my own. Dan was aware—I was confident in my ways of self-harm.

I have since stopped berating myself for why I couldn't just use my eyes a bit more back then. Why I couldn't just see into the future a bit more back then. Why I only imagined my father's ending before anything else—imagining music I'd play behind my eulogy I would one day make for him instead of seeing the small steps he'd lose instead. I feared death before losing the pieces of my father that I loved. And in those pieces that he lost, I lost in myself at the same time. I wonder if he felt a similar mourning in the way I was back then—if he looked at me in the same way I would look at him, bereft of the bond we once shared. If I could, I would have made changes—I would have made those years better for all of them. I would have sat in the passenger seat beside Flavia and nodded obediently instead of yelling at her that it was all in vain—that I needn't learn to shake hands. "It's fucking stupid, Flavia! It's just Wal-Mart!"

COMING HOME FROM The Grind, I would of course reek of cigarette smoke. And she would smell it—my mother—she would smell enough to have an asthma attack, she'd say. "Puttana! Cazzo, Stefa! You are still smoking! Naggia tutti Sant'! You better get away from me—I swear to god, you better go up to your *fucking* room!" The times she'd curse in Italian, I'd let them for the most part roll over my back and onto the floor behind me. There was a time I'd decipher the codes she used and translate them, telling all of my friends, "My mom calls me a bitch and a whore in Italian all the time. She even says the one line in Italian—'goddamn your mother'—which is sorta dumb, right? I mean, she's cursing *herself!*"

But when she switched codes, yelling curse words in English that I threw heavily onto her, those felt more piercing, more real, more tainted. And my father would open his mouth as well when we fought—but nothing would come out. His voice was stunted—it was, of course, the first that went along with numbers. Except then I needed his voice more than anything—I needed his rage, his redundant clarifications. It would take years to stop mourning his words—I would say I lamented my father's voice long before his body.

Back when he had a voice he would tell me to stop feeling guilty for my past mistakes as he held onto my shoulders and as I looked up at him. That was years ago, back when I was in the fifth and sixth grade and would tell my parents every infraction that I had committed—big or small. "Stefania, please. It's OK. I love you, you know that? I do. It will be OK," he would say to me. One evening when I was lying with my parents, I told them about something I was feeling guilty about and then followed that with a nightmare that had been troubling me. "I remember a nightmare I had once," he said. "I was swimming in the ocean. And then suddenly it got dark. I was trapped underneath a ship and I couldn't get to the surface. I couldn't breathe . . . " and the rest of his voice runs slowly across my brow.

DAN'S INITIAL FEARS proved correct—my parents found out I had cut myself again. This time, however, it was not my mother who chased me up the stairs to my room, hitting me exasperatingly—tearing things from my walls, crying and screaming at the top of her lungs. Instead, the knowledge seemed to add to her anger with me, cementing an idea she may have had in passing a year before—that I, like my father, could not be saved. Perhaps that's why her anger towards me ignited then settled, remaining at a constant flame.

I had betrayed her by hurting myself again. It was a betrayal of her trust, I realized as my father quietly walked down the stairs to the basement, where I sat in front of a computer screen. I was crying, heatedly like my mother, though it was in remembering her forgiveness of me a year before that sent me over the edge. Back then, she had screamed and fought against my actions until she realized it wouldn't change things with me—that I needed more than her fury could grant me. It took just the setting of the sun for her to forgive me—for her to kiss me goodnight as she went to bed. She would not forgive me so easily this time—the chances of her pardoning me for what I had done—again—lay in tear-filled puddles by her feet.

"Stefania," my father said, his hands in his lap.

"Dad—stop. Go upstairs. Leave me alone," I continued. I was playing solitaire and trying to focus only on the cards, trying to imagine that what was happening wasn't—again.

"I just don't understand," he continued. His speech came out fluidly, almost steadily.

"Dad—I swear. Just stop. It was a mistake."

"Why? Why do you do it?" He was staring at me. I could feel it. But I wouldn't tear my eyes away from that computer. I could hear her upstairs though, cussing and cursing me. But he was doing it his way—the old way, I remembered. The way he always seemed to do back when I was younger. He was trying to talk with me, trying to understand me, to find a way to fix me.

"Dad—Stop! JUST GO UPSTAIRS!" I screamed, though I didn't want to. I didn't want to yell at my father, who I knew didn't understand the half of it. I had hurt him, yes, but I didn't feel remorse. Not then.

"You promise me? It's the last time?" He asked. He was actually going to take my word for it. He was going to believe me if I said I would stop. He had faith in me. He, for a moment, believed that I could change. Was it because he still believed that he could get better? Because he must have not left the house that day. He was probably still in his clothing from the morning after my mother had showered, shaved and dressed him. He had probably watched television without pause, again thinking things could change with him as well. He had even started asking me about working at Wal-Mart. As a door greeter. The job that was reserved for the old people who stood in front of the automatic doors, meeting and greeting customers hour after hour. I had asked my mom why he couldn't try at least—even if only for a few hours a week. But she had told me no; he would lose his pension, his disability. He couldn't even sign his name—how would he be able to return to work?

That night I told my father I wouldn't hurt myself again, I lied. My father would again reach out to me later, yet he would resemble my mother more than himself, his *old* self. Though even my mother would never have done what he did.

No one was home but my father and me and my mother. And at one point, somehow, cutting and smoking and any number of things I was doing upset them and set *him* over the edge. He began hitting me and chased me up the stairs. I made it to my room much faster than him.

"Naggia DIO! Naggia la Madonna! 'Gia Crist!!!" He bellowed as he came towards me, holding a knife in his hand.

"Cut me!! CUT ME, STEFANIA!" He ran towards me with his hand out in front of him. His hand that held the knife grew white and strained.

I ran to the corner of my room, horrified, trembling, screaming at him— "Dad! Stop it! Stop it, dad!!" But his rage was unfiltered by a mind that was loosened, bored and angry.

The vein in his forehead, his reddening skin and his clenched teeth were reminiscent of the times he would lose control with my mother. He had never been this crazed or animal-like. His voice cracked as he growled. He grabbed me by my shoulders—"This! This is what you want!"

I didn't know how to respond or how to react. So I just cried and stared at him. Until finally, his body relaxed, he left defeated; left me, defeated.

Chapter 11

The glare of the sun through my window tore my eyes apart as I tried in vain to shut them, trying hard to fall asleep against the backdrop of that morning we drove to Pacentro. Eventually, I gave up and watched the clouds speckle the sky and the flashes of cars that we passed quickly by on that narrow highway. I looked out at the mountains, the trees that carpeted the peaks from a distance and the shadows that played on my fears as my feet edged ever closer to the small blue luggage where sat the urn of my father's ashes.

It lay right beside my left foot, and for the beginning of the drive I managed to avoid the luggage with every ounce of strength in me. Even when my mother kept the wooden box atop her dresser in her bedroom, I made sure to stay clearly away from it—yet she often asked me to look at it to see how beautiful it was. To come to terms with it.

I still heard my mother every now and then trying to talk to Zio Marco. Though I could not hear her words exactly, as I was listening to music, to a CD I cannot still remember. I would catch Zio Marco responding at times, his voice deep and strong against my mother's. Had Nicole been beside me, she would have slept for time with her own headphones securely in place. She would have been rustled awake by her spirit telling her we were approaching—that the town was not too far away. Though she wasn't with me then, I felt her there beside me and I imagined she was happy alone with Flavia.

For me, it was as if I was simply there for the moment, at least, to take notes of everything around me. Even then, I knew the drive we were taking was important—knowing I would want to remember, *need* to remember later.

It was tormenting, to say the least. Sitting still, taking note after note of what I saw, felt and understood to be temporary—looking out the window offered me a sliver of peace knowing the sky wouldn't leave; it would stay the same forever.

FLAVIA HAD STAYED behind in 2001, having what Linda and Nick Rallo would call her "Summer of Flavia." In between interning at Boeing, she'd sunbathe outside, pass many splendid hours with the Rallos and just enjoy herself finally, in an empty house. For the rest of us, even just the flight to Rome seemed to resemble the entirety of the summer through its contrast from the year prior. My father's depression and his depleting mind were taking great chunks of his personality and smashing his old self into jagged and restless pieces. The moments of him sitting still and calm were becoming vastly fewer. At this time, he had been living with dementia for four years. He was fifty-one years old.

Boarding the plane that day, my mother quickly made room for him beside her. We were able to board with the travelers with small children after my mother told them all he had Alzheimer's disease and needed extra help. She would tell people this about him whenever the need arose, but she always dropped her voice several notches lower, trying to keep this fact away from him.

I slipped by them unnoticed as my mother fumbled hurriedly through her bags.

"OK Giovann—take this pillow," my mother instructed my father, as she took another two from beside her and propped them around him tightly, as though he were packaged between cushion and skin. "Do you want something to drink? Do you have to go to the bathroom? Are you OK? Do you need anything?"

He looked at her and shook his head, barely breathing a quick, "No."

Meanwhile, I was having issues with Nicole—"Nic, why do you have to put all your crap on my side of the seat?" I looked at her angrily as she looked up at me in her little barrettes.

"Stefania, caz—will you leave her alone? She's only ten, you know!" Mom was always listening, always a hawk watching, waiting.

"I'm sorry, Stef." Nicole said apologetically, as she tried to move things. I felt guilty but said nothing. Closing my eyes, I waited for departure.

GREETING PEOPLE IN the town, I watched as my father acted much more subdued. When he did attempt to blend in, I can see all he had left to do was try and mimic my mother.

"Ciao!! Giovanni! Enida!!" Franca exclaimed as we approached her bar later that evening, after my mother had showered herself then my father. Nicole and I followed closely behind.

"Stefa!! Nicole! Venite qui!" Franca told us as she reached towards us, kissing us on either cheek. I spotted Claudia and quickly hugged her as well. The year before we had been inseparable—this year, though, simply in the greeting I felt a thicker air around me, and it was hard to act comfortable—normal, even—though I couldn't reason what normal would look like at that moment. Surely, it wasn't the way we stood there. I hoped in that instant of greeting they had noticed he wasn't well. Maybe it was pity I was after or understanding even. Whatever it was though, he was a different man than before and he stood awkwardly between knowing and forgetting and more awkwardly still, within the definition of Alzheimer's disease. Most people with that disease could fake it more—the content he did utter would just be off. But not him—if he could form words, however sparse, it would be enough. Simply being able to hear him would have masked whatever foul content or misappropriated word he may or may not have uttered.

"Perche' non venite qua a mangiare una pizza stasera?" Franca asked my mom and dad—knowing how much they did enjoy eating the pizza at her bar. Multiple times a week the year before they had sat to eat dinner beside her and others outside. She was hoping they could get started right away.

My father stood smiling at Franca with his arms resting above his backside, embracing his hands one within the other. He curled the corner of his lip a bit, almost sarcastically, as though he were telling a joke with a facial gesture. Or he stood smiling like he was in on the joke, the story, anything at all really. By then, he seemed aware that if he tried to speak, he'd fail. He depended then, on hints and subtleties that I picked up on painfully.

"Mo' dobbiamo salutare fratem'. Domani sera, pero, sara' meglio. 'Ua bon?" My mom said, as she looked over at Nicole, me, and finally at my dad. She had promised her brother we'd come by later that evening and eat with his family. Tomorrow—tomorrow night it seemed would fare better.

"OK—" Franca said, as she embraced my parents again, kissing them once on each cheek.

"Ciao," said my father quickly; it was the only word he managed to utter. He nodded for emphasis as he turned towards my mother and followed her outside.

Outside, my mom took hold of his arm, pushing him slightly forward as we walked towards her brother's home through Vico Diritto. His slow shuffles were exasperating her. Everywhere we went, he always lagged behind.

Finally, we reached the house. I stepped over dried bits of cat droppings around the front stoop and pressed the doorbell.

"Look, Stef! Pasta for the cats!" Nicole exclaimed. I followed her gaze down to a few bowls with scraps of pasta inside. I imagined Zia Franca affectionately taking the day's remnants of food and putting them outside for all of her cats. Even the strays would gather around the food, the same strays who decorated the streets of the town like the Cat's Meow Village that adorned the tops of the doorframes in our home in Missouri.

We heard the door above us on the balcony squeak open and her light footsteps coming to a stop at the railing. "Eh!! Benvenuti!!" Zia Franca yelled down to us. Dropping her head over, her long, stringy, light brown hair fell in front of her face, covering her glasses. "Mo vengo!" We heard her shoes clattering against the stairs seconds after we heard the buzz of the door, allowing us to push our way into the foyer.

I can see time in frames that remain imprinted on the years I look back, remembering the specific moments of his forgetting take form. At dinner, as we all sat together, my father took his knife and fork in his hands and scraped them delicately over the meat. I'm sure it must have been aniello or bistecca and I'm sure he was eager and yet dreading that moment when, without a word, my mother reached to his plate and began cutting his meat for him. As she did in the States, so she would do in Pacentro. She would cut his food for him for the remainder of the trip, never looking up to meet anyone's gaze, never saying a word to my father. Just knowing that it had to be done. She had no choice—and neither did he.

Pacentro's air and sunlight hit my parents' spirits hard, especially my mother who had decided to breathe new life into her desperation. From all the days and afternoons spent lying on her bed mourning her husband who had not yet left her, her hopes were mainly quashed. From the doctors' perspectives, the symptoms would only progress. Even if the dementia my father had was not indeed Alzheimer's disease, it was still leaving her crushed within its wake. So having been raised in a town where sheep are still herded, pasta e fagioli still eaten in cantinas, and homemade olive oil given out to neighbors in old glass or plastic bottles, my mother returned to faith. Perhaps more faith is what she needed—maybe it's what we all needed. And what better way to jumpstart faith than going on a pilgrimage in hopes of a miracle.

I didn't want to go—I told my friends and my cousin as much, even begged my mother to just let me stay behind. Nicole, too, couldn't stand the thought of leaving behind her friends, her bicycle that a year before had been the cause of her hitting her head against the cement tunnel within the labyrinth of our section of town—La Guardiola—and needing stitches. It didn't phase her though, as she still enjoyed wandering the old cobblestones like her mother had, like her father.

But we went anyway. On a sunny afternoon, my mother drove us down Monte Morrone, clear across La Valle Peligna. She drove for hours on the autostrada heading towards Puglia, into a province of Foggia to a town called San Giovanni Rotondo. It was here that Padre Pio lived for fifty-two years—here, in the town, that like Pacentro, is set within the mountains, sitting gracefully within a valley surrounded by majestic mountains that herald their might. Both towns, differing in just about eighty meters in elevation, have sat engulfed within their own history, peopled century after century, flourishing, surviving.

In this way, we were like the town we ascended, parking in a crowded lot reserved for tourists—or for those seeking a cure, a miracle, or a place to worship. I feel the heat again like I did in Rome when I try to remember the specifics outside. I only hear the gravel beneath my shoes and people surrounding me. I remember there was a line we stood in—or maybe, instead, we waited inside the Santa Maria delle Grazie, Our Lady of Grace Church. Within that Church is the shrine of Padre Pio. And just who was this man?—I knew very little as we walked within the last shreds of my mother's hope.

Today I have his picture on my wall. Padre Pio, in brown gloves, the tips of the finger holes cut away. His white beard contrasts with his salt and pepper, close cropped hair. He holds one hand in the air as though to make the sign of the cross with the side of his right palm. His face is contorted in pain and reverie; he is no doubt praying, concentrating, feeling blessed with his connection to Christ.

I have his picture on my bedroom wall today because a year after we visited his tomb, walking the narrow hallways, looking in on his old room, the clothes he wore and saw the objects he touched—he was ordained a Saint. And before this Saint, I stood beside my parents and we prayed for a miracle—for my father to get well.

But we didn't get the miracle we had prayed for—that we had traveled miles for from our own mountain village to another. And in that travel, we didn't see that there, in the Piazza del Popolo in Pacentro, stood a church that held more chance of a miracle than the one we had visited. Among our past and present and the future we feared stood the connective piece of our lineage—The Church of the Santa Maria della Misercordia, the Our Lady of Mercy Church. It was there, shortly after my father's birth in his home on that small side road, down where the moths hang on cement and stone and voices of children still bounce in corners, where stray cats mingle in the day. It was in that Church of Mercy that the late Don Giuseppe, affectionately known by the townsfolk as Don Peppe, baptized my father. Don Peppe died in 2009, after living almost ninety-three years in that town, as the priest who helped those in need, offering condolences, love, and most of all, hope.

I remember each time I'd pass Don Peppe; his crooked back bent forward, his pale head burning in the sun beneath his light and wispy white hair. He wore glasses, round ones that still allowed the brilliance of his eyes to show through. I imagine them blue—though I never spoke so closely to him and studied him. I only remember the path he walked and the reactions left behind him. I only see, now, moments of my father kissing Don Peppe on either cheek, embracing him and introducing him to me as a child.

And it was again Don Peppe who gave my mother her first communion, who stood before the light from the wooden altar again when she was twenty and my father twenty-eight. Don Peppe, who married them, sent them out the doorway of the church, to the early autumn air where they would walk among the townspeople to continue their marriage celebrations and continue on their path as husband and wife, father and mother.

It was this church in this town that would bring us more hope than anywhere else. Because this church was our church and this town was our town. The strength of our love and the resilience of our family were in each glint of sun and graceful speck of dust.

WE WOULDN'T REALIZE this though. I don't believe anyone ever does, really—no one ever really gets the point of it all or sees the larger picture when you're stuck in it knee deep and dragging. That is what our summer was. My mother went out most days, talking with friends, spending time with the ones she grew up with—gauging, again, the pluses and minuses of living there. And my father, what was becoming of him, was like a stench that hung too low to the ground. I was suffocated by his depression and the change I saw in his spirit. He didn't arrive that summer like that—at least I hadn't noticed if he had. He showed just hints here and there back at home—he was more withdrawn. He tried to speak less at home. But sometimes, I remember, I did see him sad and I did feel sorry for him. I thought that he could get out of his despair though—but why would I of all people have expected more of him? Again, I wouldn't understand why until much later. I was struggling against feeling anger at him and everyone else while he often didn't bother moving from the living room for more than a meal if he even chose to eat at all.

One afternoon, while my mother was away talking to a friend in the piazza and Nicole was sitting playing Tetris by the window, I made lunch. And I made that lunch with the intention of forcing it down my father's throat. He had spent quite a bit of time up in his bedroom and he wouldn't get out of bed. It was going on a day and a half of him lying there. And with the afternoon heat as it was he must have been dying—must have been needlessly suffering. And so I made lunch and when it was done I went upstairs to get him and bring him downstairs. When I reached the door, I found it locked. He wouldn't answer my initial calls until I banged on the door and he meakly told me, "No."

Suddenly I had had enough. In the way that my mother had enough when she drove us into Puglia, to her last chance of hope, I decided to write a friend a letter but never send it. I followed the cue of my father's own hopelessness as he lay in bed on the other side of the wall I sat against. I heaved with silent tears and my hands shook as I wrote a three-page letter, in blue ink.

"*I am feeling more and more like shit,*" I started bluntly. "*Everyday, I feel myself slipping away. I feel the dread of returning to my old ways. This fear chokes me, but I'm too weak to fight it off.*" It took all I had to keep myself from cutting, from screaming. I thought about how I missed my friends back home, most of all Dan—and how at least at home, I could get my mind off things. I wasn't completely surrounded by my family.

I then began writing about the lunch I had just made *"to keep me busy and shield the fact that my dad stayed in bed for a day and a half without eating."* And my tone shifts as I reveal that *"his reason was so he could die."* My mother, before leaving that day, had *"informed him that that was the slowest way and wouldn't work."*

I can see myself digging the pen even deeper into the page as I continue, *"This isn't about my father. It has nothing to do with the fact that he can't put his own shirt on by himself, that he eats with the skill of a five year old—cutting his bread with a knife and fork. Nor does it have to do with the fact that I screamed at him to take his medicine—to wake up this morning—and not once have I comforted him as he lay there—anticipating his death, tasting his hope—salivating on the thought."* The speed at which I'm writing seems to diminish as I continue: *"No. I can't deal with him. Guilt stabs my every limb when I look at him. He's my father, was. Now he's just a child in a dying man's body."*

It's at this point in the letter when perhaps my father begins to stir. *"I miss him. I miss my father."* It's when I start with these confessions that I imagine he resolves to sit up. *"I miss that man who would come home just as my mom was putting the dinner on the table. I miss that man who I'd run to when he'd open the door. I'd scream '1,2,3' and leap into his arms and he'd set me down, smiling. I miss playing foosball with him—trying so hard to beat him. We'd start off with 'just one more game' then three, then seven. I miss that man who'd answer all my questions with excessive details—making sure I understood through and through what I wanted to know. I miss his laugh. I miss his voice. I miss my dad."*

I had never, until then, listed the parts of my father that I missed. I had never, until that night, relived those moments that were so tender and so cherished—in haste. Instead, I saved the moments of melancholy for my window seat where they would just come gliding through and over me until I was completely numb.

ON THE OTHER side of the wall, my father's steps to his door are slow as I grow angrier writing the letter: "*What the fuck did I ever do—did anyone in my immediate family ever do? That's what everyone always asks, right? When their life is in the shit hole? . . . I don't know who I am, what I want. Fuck all I've done—screw the messes I've gotten into. Let me erase the memories that haunt my mind and maybe then I could sit by myself for once in peace. Because day after day, I'm being beaten by my own mind . . . I'm slipping, returning back to what I was or what I am or who I was made to be . . . Maybe this is just a hump, just one of those 'low spells' I get. But it is all too real to be just that. It is all here and I'm living and breathing every inch of it . . .*"

He wasn't mine any longer. And not once did I lie beside him. I wrote it. It must be true. I can't believe I didn't lie with him that morning I yelled at him to take his medicine. I can't believe I didn't hold him, take his shoulders in my hands and shake him. I didn't let my own tears mix with his own like his had done with mine.

"What are you doing?" he asked me, almost normally, as he suddenly appeared in my open doorway.

"Nothing—I'm just writing," I told him, my eyes red and my cheeks still hot.

He nodded slightly and stood a minute longer. Maybe he knew I was crying. Maybe he knew he had upset me when he told me he wanted to die. Maybe he knew I missed him more in that moment than I had yet allowed myself.

But instead of asking him, I swallowed my curiosity. "I'm getting allergies," I said, as I raised my hands to my eyes and caught the tears before they fell.

Chapter 12

I never did see my father walking around the town as he had the year before. Never did I pass by him in my cousin Claudio's car as we mainly sat in silence, again listening to a heated song by a band whose anger seemed to match my own. I don't believe I ever did see him again standing by himself, staring into the Valle Peligna as he had the year before when I turned away abruptly and continued the drive into town with my cousin.

Instead, that year I closed my own mouth much like he did—and tried, just like my father—to fit in. I would sit on steps and stoops within the town with Claudio, with Claudia, and others. Michele and his cousin Giuseppe came to be steady members of the group. And it would be me trying to sit a bit closer beside Giuseppe, and trying to keep my eyes on him that seemed to take much of my thinking away that summer.

Out on the balcony, I could feel my father behind the white curtains of the doors to his bedroom as I sat with my back against him. My legs hanging between the railings, I'd feel the summer wind while he lay with the windows closed behind me. I didn't think to open those doors, to knock and have him greet me, invite him outside along with me. I didn't think to ask him how it felt back in the seventies when he stood below me on the winding pathway those runners took on the Corsi degli Zingari. I didn't ask him if he remembered yelling after them, clapping for someone in particular or for no one at all, feeling excitement growing in his body that moved gracefully among his friends.

I just let him lie there while I basked in the sun, smoking when my mother was away. I learned I could smoke while "staying with" my father—he would never think it was me or wouldn't know how to approach me, let alone rebuke me.

And on that balcony I would come to realize something strange, something exciting and something different. It took just a few weeks for me to realize I was in love that summer—in love with a boy from Pacentro.

MY FATHER USED to love to jog. He'd run on weekends in the late morning with shorts on and usually, an old tee shirt from Mexico or any other summer trip we may have gone on. He usually wore a baseball cap as well—again, it was usually from Mexico. One in particular that he loved to wear was neon pink with "Mexico" written glaringly across the front. I came to love that hat of his, the baseball cap with the flat-as-a-board bill that he wore atop his sweaty head. It enlivened his runs, I think. I think he favored his pink cap above all the others.

I tried jogging with my dad one summer. We were vacationing in Puerto Vallarta my spring break of sixth grade—two years before he was diagnosed. I ran beside him as he'd tell me, "In through your nose, Stefania. Out through your mouth—like this," as he exaggeratingly took deep gulps of air into his nostrils, letting it out again through his o-shaped lips, sounding like wind through an open car window.

Inevitably, I would stop—complain of chest pain and no breath. He would stop with me and then we'd start again. I dreaded going further, knowing I'd have to run back, while he kept his head up straight, his eyes focused. He kept such good form that each time he'd turn his head away from me, holding one nostril and blowing out the other, I'd hardly even notice. "Dad—did you just blow your nose on your finger?" And he'd laugh at me as I cringed in disgust.

It was Flavia who got the running genes and later Nicole. Flavia often jogged with him—up until he wouldn't be able to keep up with her. She remembers the sudden change in him; one of the first signs was the running. He'd be the one to fall behind, to stop, to give up.

And he would also blow his nose any which way he wanted—often right on Flavia's side. I don't believe he even noticed.

He jogged that summer in Pacentro like he did the others. Though that year it was different. My mom would have helped him into his shorts, laid out his socks and tied his shoes. She would have reminded him to use the bathroom before he left—would have feigned relief perhaps that he was going out alone. Because she knew he shouldn't.

And on a particular day that summer my father left the house. He would have passed by Maria and Giuseppina as they sat on wooden house chairs outside their front doors. They would have greeted one another as he would've started off. Slowly he'd begin, jogging carefully on the uneven ground, through the portals with the fresco of the Madonna painted before my father was but a thought in the wind that carried the voices of the villagers through the open windows in the town.

But suddenly his running may have altered and he would have forgotten the rhythm of his breathing—in through your nose, out through your mouth. Yet he would still ascend the mountain he knew well—at that time, he seemed to know it better than himself.

Back on Via Guardiola, my mother would start feeling anxious. In fact, she was always nervous when he ventured outside her vision and that day he left to go jogging—he took longer than he should have to return.

I don't know how much time passed before she called him—I don't even remember the day it happened. I don't know if my mother went to ask her friend in person or on the phone, but she did it just the same. She waited at home while her friend got into his carozzino, a small three-wheeled truck, and drove up the mountain, following the lead of townspeople who had seen him.

He drove up past the steep turns and farther past the trees beneath which I would sit with friends and later park with Giuseppe alone at night.

If I were upstairs asleep I wouldn't have heard my mother pacing the living room downstairs, finally shutting the windows before she left to wait outside. I wouldn't have heard her telling Maria and Giuseppina that she was worried about her husband, who an hour or more before had gone out running and hadn't come back.

My mother's friend would finally come to an area up the mountain where our neighbors, the Bussis, kept a stable open for visitors in the summer. There he would find my father, panting near the horses, drinking water from a fountain.

He stopped running and I didn't notice. He was getting sicker now, as I sat below them in our house that summer she would bathe and dress him. I would sit entranced by the shadows from the wood-paneled living room as I sat on the soft, velvety sofa beside the breeze from the window that stood slightly ajar. Above the fireplace stood a ledge with photos framed along its length. In them all were the signs of my parent's love. I breathed in a sigh that may have matched his own as he sat with her upstairs. The two of them upstairs at that moment would have been so very different from the memories they shared of my mother turning slyly towards my father. It must have been a clear and sunny day in the square when she asked him, "Mi compri delle noccioline?" and he buying, in turn, those peanuts for her lofty flirtations and his thirsty spirit the first time they touched.

GIUSEPPE AND I became friends when it was warm outside. The sun was shining on all the stones and the water as it spilled from the fountain in the Piazza del Popolo. I would see the scene in my mind as clear as I would the day he left me, putting a cassette tape in my hand and I looking down, spilling forth a final goodbye of tears that fall harder than the rain.

But that would come to happen only after I gave my heart to him, gave my everything—and most importantly, my hope. I realize now how that girl of seventeen must have seemed to him: scared, angry, and lonely. I see now that I turned to a love of a different kind when I had nothing else to hold onto.

"Sono un fantasma," he told me as he walked me home one evening. I had been sitting in the Piazza Iaringhi, on a few stairs that led up into a building. Claudia, Michele, and Giuseppe were there. Others sat amongst us but my memory only highlights the true pieces that help to tell the story.

"Devo andare a casa," I told them all as I stood up. It was nearly midnight and my mother would be home waiting for me. She didn't change much from her American self that summer in regard to my curfews and her evening breath analysis. So when it was time, I regretfully gathered up my things, put a piece of gum in my mouth to mask the smell of cigarettes and beer and said goodbye.

"Aspetta, Stefa. Ti accompagno," Giuseppe said as he quickly caught up to me. He wanted to walk with me, and as I felt us growing closer as friends, I welcomed him. We would often spend the evenings together with all our friends, including his cousin and my own. For about a week, I had been "dating" his cousin, who had kissed me suddenly in the street. His cousin had loved me in the way you care deeply for someone—mi voleva bene. But it wasn't love, romantic love—amare. I don't believe that was even a question. Yet I had consented to be with him, allowing him to treat me as a girlfriend, though lightly, kissing lightly, holding lightly. But Giuseppe was always in the back of my mind, and as they say, Giuseppe came and swept me away.

We passed by his house on Vico Diritto and he kept walking. I realized he was going to walk the whole way with me. We mainly walked in silence, yet every so often we'd say a word or two, though I can't hear the words as they were. Only three remain from that evening. And he spoke them slyly, almost seductively. "Sono un fantasma."

"Come?" I asked him incredulously. We were nearing my house, standing outside the Bussi's home, beneath a lone yellow light. "Sono un fantasma" he said again.

And I laughed somewhat, giving him a look that at once said "you're crazy," and then nervously dissolved into not understanding.

But he just looked at me, smiling slightly. The light from the small bulb above us lit his brown eyes; his dark brown hair nearly glowed. I wanted to continue asking him how and why he believed he was a ghost. I wanted to tell him how I watched his breathing in his chest, his sweat on his forehead beneath his bangs that he often brushed up into his hair, how I could almost taste his sweet and sour mountain air smell.

But that was before he became my definition of freedom with my face towards the sky in his blue car, letting the air pat my face, powdering my pale skin that I kept behind a layer of mourning. It was in this air that I found my love, my medicine, which would be the first in turn for him. Yet unlike him, I was needing him, I was in need of him. And he, unknowingly, probably, fell into me thinking he had a rope he could use to climb out.

AND IT STARTED just like that. It came to me just so—just like the wind could carry with it just enough cold air to ease the heat inside our house during the long and restless days. I would go outside in the evenings to find my cousin Claudio and see Giuseppe in the mix as well. His eyes would be there to greet me and his silence in the words he spoke behind the ones I heard is what gripped me, and I looked at him and in an instant I could feel myself again living, again reliving.

Eventually he kissed me but I can't for the life of me remember when or remember how or remember where we stood. Was it that night, one of the first he took the chance to be near me, when he told me he was a ghost and scoffed? And I knew in a way he was right, and I knew beyond reason that he would be right.

No, I believe the first time was at La Furnacella, a restaurant and hotel that sits up away from Pacentro, up the road that leads up the mountain. Outside, there is a wraparound seating area where the views of Pacentro are at their finest. Especially at night, when the lights within the town illuminate the castle towers in shades of orange and yellow. On that particular evening, I had gone inside to use the bathroom—mainly just to get away for a moment. I was sitting at a table with Giuseppe, his cousin, my cousin and others, and left them all so that I could gather my thoughts.

The bathroom was in a separate room. On one side of the wall was a sink and a mirror, where I stood before two doors separating two stalls—one for women and the other for men.

And I still feel my body tense, my excitement overflowing through my eyes that screamed in joy as I saw Giuseppe walk in. We stood beside the same sink pretending to wash our hands, but really just using it as an excuse to touch one another innocently. We stopped and moved closer—our heads tilting, our eyes closing—as the door opened and his cousin entered.

Everyone left shortly afterwards and Giuseppe's cousin was the last to go. They would later argue outside Zia Franca's house—and I would hide away in my house on my balcony.

And that was our dramatic beginning, that summer my father stopped running up the mountain.

Chapter 13

We decided to keep our relationship a secret, Giuseppe and I. I started feeling nervous and too anxious going out at night with Claudio and his friends. My *friends* became estranged from me and Giuseppe's cousin, the one I had been seeing, couldn't stand to look at me. Since I already had such anxiety and depression on my own, the situation didn't seem to help me at all, but instead, made me feel far worse than I needed to at all. I was just a girl of seventeen and Giuseppe would be turning nineteen that winter. Yet I believed there was another force inherent to that love, a connection to my past—and I came to realize this in nothing more than his words, through his voice.

Looking back now, it is all so clear, as though the scenes were written down, from the moments I would reach my hand for his as he'd drive me to Sulmona, to the ways his lips parted before speaking.

He'd borrow his father's blue car, and we'd drive down the mountain and into Sulmona, drinking wine and basking in the love that soon engulfed us. Gaeta was where he would take me—up above a massive flight of stairs were seats and tables along the outside of a small bar. I still don't know if that is the name of the bar or simply a word used to describe the hangout that teenagers in that area would go to. In the Piazza Iaringhi, he would park and we would walk hand in hand across the large square, where there, too, sat a fountain, much larger than the one in our Piazza del Popolo. In Pacentro, it takes less than a minute or so to cross, save for the intersections of hellos and minimal conversations. Across the Piazza Garibaldi and in Sulmona as a whole, one could walk in tranquility or may suddenly be stopped for pleasantries or on a whim by a fellow Pacentrano who might be in town for shopping. And perhaps because it is the birthplace of Ovid, I realize even more the change I felt grow inside me. It was not despair, for once, but hope I felt when I kissed him, held him and loved him.

On our final night together, we sat beneath a streetlamp on a quiet and empty road in Sulmona. Parking, perhaps like they had parked—my parents—beside the same trees and the same stones. My father may have laughed as he bought her those peanuts, may have scoffed, and later may have driven her below the town, across the fields that swept by in the wind and then they may have settled beneath a streetlamp and embraced.

GIUSEPPE HAD A habit of staring at me, into my eyes, for long bouts of time. And in exchange for those times where I felt he was really seeing me, really seeing into me, I would look at him as well. And that last night was no exception. I gave my entire sense of self into that stare that I shared with him, telling him with my silence that for once I felt happy, felt complete. That I felt hope was certain and sealed in me that evening when we shared one seat and I leaned against him in his scratchy sweater. And then he whispered it into my ear and I sat up and watched him tell me again. "Ti amo, Stefania," and it wasn't love, his love that he was telling me he had for me that made my heart as full as it had ever been. It was the way he said my name, the way the words came out so wonderfully familiar that made it hard for me to turn away. It was his wonted intonation of my name and all the rest of the questions, the statements and proclamations that he made to me beneath that streetlamp, that swayed me and moved me. I could do without their meaning, only I couldn't live without their sound.

After we realized the time and knew we needed to soon turn away and head back up to Pacentro, we sat just a moment longer and let the smoke escape from our lungs and our mouths from cigarettes on which we'd written *I love you* in both our languages, listening to a tape of Smashing Pumpkins he loved and I loved in return. Gabriella Ferri maybe, or Mia Martini, perhaps, even sang to them as my father's beard bristled against my mother's soft cheeks and her curls that indelibly touched his heart.

It seemed that I had found my father again but only as a young man, who felt and saw the same life that he had then been leaving. And so I loved Giuseppe. I loved him with such strength that when it would eventually leave me, I would barely be able to open my eyes to my father's last stages without feeling the pang of a love I lost that promised me an end to all of that suffering.

I WAS STRUGGLING to keep my foot at a distance from the blue luggage—keeping my torso bent just slightly so my legs and feet would be kept safely in the other direction. But, gradually, my anxiety was lifting and a cool and pleasant calm began to surround me. One by one, I felt each joint in my body release as they were all clenched so tightly. My neck and shoulders felt as though they were floating separately—while each of my fingers extended just slightly, feeling as though they were submerged in unruffled waters.

And so too did my breathing change, growing in intensity and depth, from into my nose, down into my belly and out again through my mouth, gliding smoothly like a wisp of cotton. So amid the humming of my uncle's car, I moved my foot to sit against the urn of my father's ashes.

It happened almost suddenly, right after a lull in my breathing, when every ounce of me felt still and complacent. I did so without thought or fear, just certainty that I needed to be as near to his body—or what remained of it—as possible. It would be the last time I could touch him, though through a box and the added confines of the blue luggage, it was as though I had suddenly grasped my father's hand. And so I made sure not to move an inch, so as to keep his hand held tightly in mine.

I stared out my window and waited for changing thoughts and feelings to swim about in my mind. It certainly did pain me, knowing this was as close as I would ever come again. That my father now remained in a wooden box with his name engraved with the dates of his living made me shiver, but it warmed me just the same. Where he lay now was body and air inside an urn whose mere vicinity to my foot made my breathing sparse and my heart ache with a weight I hadn't felt before. But oddly enough, I breathed freely when I finally gave in and let my foot rest against his urn.

Meanwhile, the Appennini Mountains surrounded us on all sides of that small car. We could now spot various small mountain towns that lay indiscriminately among the peaks and pockets of the mountains. The road was beginning to be more variable, every so often bringing forth a guardrail on either side which separated us from the cliffs that stood gaping on either side. Then just as quickly, we neared a tunnel cut directly into the side of the mountain. Inside, the lights above us became one streaming line of yellow light, the air whipping against our car and the inner walls of the mountain, and the silence that ensued stood in stark contrast to when we'd finally emerge and be met once again with the sun, the Appennini Mountains, and the darkened faces of my family I could not see before.

My mother's jaw seemed lax and I could see the bags beneath her tired eyes as she sat. She kept her gaze firm and steady towards the road in front of her. She didn't flinch from the weight of sleep that I'm sure she must have felt, and I wonder how truly scared or anxious she may have been. Or any of the times, really, before that day we drove there. I wanted to rub her back as she sat there alone beside her brother. I wanted to sit beside her, take her arms in mine and hold her.

But that was never really my mother's way—she finds it easier to express anything other than mushy affection, as she may think of it. Yes, she would hold my hand often, but I came to think she delighted in being angry, in finding reasons and ways to push me away. That night I came back from my last evening with Giuseppe, she had met me at the door with—"Puttana!! Did you give him a nice present!? Eh? Troia!" Her branding me a whore stung worse than if she had slapped me squarely on the cheek. I was several hours late and we were to leave at daybreak the next day, so her anger was expected. Her fear, I realized later—for me, her daughter—was also a part of her delirium, but I hadn't cared. I only cared about myself and my then breaking-heart. I slept on the balcony that evening or tried to. I stared up at the moon, looked out to the Furnacella—whose lights stayed on throughout the night. I tried to melt atop the concrete of the floor and fall like water down the sides.

Everyday I wore Giuseppe's wooden beaded necklace he had given me. It was my senior year in high school and I was in love—and the necklace was my only keepsake. Meanwhile, my mother and I didn't speak for weeks after we got home. Nicole, though, would often sit with me and listen to me cry and pine for Giuseppe. She was so sweetly innocent to how I had frightened my mother and how I was so involved with just my own despair.

One afternoon, my father and I sat at the kitchen table. I can see the light through the window of the sliding doors that open to our deck. My father sits in a short sleeve shirt as I look at him through watery eyes and tell him how in love I am with a boy from Pacentro.

"Dad—I'm going to move there. After school. I'm gonna teach English and maybe live in Sulmona," I told him. I was giddy with dreams for my future and Giuseppe's. And so I shared my life plans on an afternoon with my dementia-ridden father who managed to ask me, smiling, "will you marry him?" And I said I would. I felt no guilt nodding my head emphatically and with conviction saying yes.

I didn't think that my father felt a slight bit of sadness because unlike my mother, my father was quite affectionate. And as a child I had loved it. When company would be over, I'd hear him often talking, laughing—making them all laugh in turn. In the kitchen, he would sit with his legs parted slightly, his arms crossed, his head resting slightly on his hand. I would watch him from the doorway, seeing the light shine through his eyes and the lenses of his glasses. "Stefania," he'd say, "come here."

I'd push the wall away from me and hop towards him. He'd move his chair away from the table and motion for me to sit on his legs.

"You're my little girl," he'd tell me, as he'd brush my hair away from my cheeks. I'd smile fully and nestle further onto his lap. "She promised me she'd never get married," he said once to company as I proudly nodded in agreement.

But when I told him I would indeed break that promise, he had just looked wistfully at me, looking more content than angry—less jealous than pleased.

I STOPPED HEARING from Giuseppe soon after I received his second letter in October. I'd lie on my floor, his letters and his necklace splayed out around me. I knew then that he had failed me. I was heartbroken thinking he could have been my cure. He could have been the eyes I needed to look at me as though I were everything. His eyes were, I imagined, the eyes that would undoubtedly make me smile with a force so pure. He had become my image of hope, a dream I had and had since lost.

But all I had was this man's "ti amo" that I no longer heard. And I never even got to know why. I just received a silence from the other end of his phone that kept ringing and a space left empty in the mail. I sought closure when I'd go to therapy, telling my doctor, pleading with her to give me a magic cure to make me feel OK. I couldn't feel OK—I felt worse than I had ever felt before.

My hope had failed me when he said he loved me; that he'd wait for me and call me and write to me—and then he stopped. He stopped suddenly, not eventually. I didn't hear a strain in him or a pause or a stutter. I didn't see the love gradually leave him in stages like my father's life was then consuming.

So I grew more withdrawn and returned to therapy, like I had been going on and off since middle school. I had been on and off psychotropic drugs since my father had taught me how to drive, and I would be returning to them again.

At the same time, my mother began entrusting me to watch my father more regularly on weekends, and I would grow enraged.

"So now that Nicole is finally old enough to watch herself, I have to watch *dad*?!" I'd scream.

She'd grind her teeth in anger and chase me up the stairs—"Do you think I like this, Stefa!? Do you think I enjoy this!?"

I know I was to feel guilt when she said that and I did—I know that for sure. But when she'd leave to go to the mall, to the bookstore, to wherever she needed to go to breathe without him there as a reminder—I'd take advantage wholeheartedly. Instead of sitting beside him on the couch or offer to talk with him—*to* him, more likely—I would sit in the dark in my bedroom with headphones on or sneak out onto the deck and smoke cigarettes.

I would sit with him sparingly. When I would, I'd ask him if he wanted an ice cream or some cookies. I didn't bother telling him I was sad because I didn't want to burden him. I think he probably knew I was different—in just a look, I could see his concern. His eyebrow would bend; his eyes would squint slightly. His mouth would open slightly and I could tell he wanted to say things to me, and I can only imagine now what they would be. I like to think he may have wanted to tell me Giuseppe was just a boy—something along the lines of love hurts—maybe he'd tell me about his first love and how it ended. But I'd laugh it off in front of him and instead return to the offer of a cookie, of a snack. He loved sneaking them when my mother wasn't looking—and I loved the way his eyes lit up, the way he'd nod so eagerly as I'd get up from the couch and go get one. Because although he couldn't speak to me as a father would, his eagerness at enjoying the simple bites of a cookie alongside me would be enough for me. It would be enough because it would be all I could get.

My mother would return after he had gone up to bed. I would follow him upstairs and ask him if he needed help—though, so soon after Italy, I don't believe he needed me to undress him just yet. Instead, I'd make sure he was on his way to bed and the lights were out before I'd make my way to my room and into my closet. I'd reach for a bottle of Jack Daniels I had paid an ex-coworker to buy me and pour myself a drink.

I STARTED DRINKING alone in my bedroom not too long after we returned from Pacentro. Even just after leaving Giuseppe, I felt the pangs of my depression return and sweep over me. When I started receiving his letters, my obsession of my imagined future with him grew stronger and my unhappiness in my home increased.

Sometimes, I would sit in the dark while my parents were in the living room. I could see them clearly in my thoughts as I toasted to our miserable life that we had returned to. My mother's sanity seemed a bit depleted and her patience was growing thin. My parents were now fighting much more and they seldom left the house together during the day. That is why my mother resorted to her random nightly trips to the mall—to anywhere other than that living room or her bedroom. And my father would grow angry, spiteful—perhaps even jealous. But he'd remain, for the most part, on that recliner until sleep would finally hit him and he'd make his way slowly towards his bedroom.

So I would have my Jack Daniels on nights when I thought for sure I'd be left alone. And I'd think of how desperate everything was now becoming. And thrown atop my discontent was now the realization that I was on my own. I had loved imagining my life in the future, imagining myself with Giuseppe driving together in our black Fiat 500, living together somewhere on a vineyard in Italy.

But suddenly he was gone—in an instant, he had taken all of that away. I wasn't accustomed to that feeling of remorse. I was used to imagining the worst before having reason to do so. In my father's case, I had imagined my eulogy before he had even been a fraction of what he would become.

So on a night when my mother slept, embittered, as my father lay beside her, growing more childlike and ill, I sat alone across the hall in my bedroom. As usual, I had my headphones on while listening to some CD that I'm sure must have matched my mood. I had set the cold glass of whiskey in my lap as I stared at the tips of my toes where they rested on the window seat. Raising my eyes slowly to the branches of the trees outside, I was met with the still midnight sky. I swayed my head slowly to the music, sloshing the ice cubes around my glass. And across the hall, my mother opened her eyes.

My door rattled from her pounding fists; her screams were glass-breaking, shaking—tearing my ears with their pitch. I threw the bottle of Jack Daniel's under my bed as she unlocked my door with a bobby pin. I waited and held my breath as she swept through my room, breaking CDs, breaking photo frames and figurines, tearing posters, tearing signs. Then she turned to me as I escaped in drunkenness yet again, escaped from all sides of her hands that hit me, hard and deserved. I felt angry and guilty and deaf. My ways of coping again seemed to hurt her just as badly as my father's descent seemed to crush her. But I could control my ways, whereas he could not. I was the only one who could be blamed.

She blamed me as well for choosing drinking as my second way to cope. Her grip was firm as she swung her seventeen-year-old daughter by the hair onto her bed. "Brutta puttana! Just like my father! Sei come lui! Come mio padre!!"

I remember falling onto my bed as she left my room. I remember hearing Nicole faintly in the background, crying.

Twice I woke up—once when the light in my room from outside was gentle, baby blue and fuzzy. I looked around and thought I had dreamt it—but then I saw the devastation in my room and I quickly fell back asleep.

I awoke the second time just as my whitewashed door adorned with scraps of torn posters opened again, rattling, and slammed against the wall. I looked at her wild eyes, already dark and crazed as she said with so much malice and spite, "Look what you are doing to him. Keep it up, Stefa. Keep it up." She threw a stack of stapled paper at me and then, she left—just as suddenly.

My head, of course, was throbbing; I was sure I had large chunks of hair missing—semi-scalped perhaps, at least. I lay in bed a second longer, hearing her march down the staircase. When I finally heard her walking towards the living room, I sat up and began to read.

On the first page, I read: "Courage in Caregiving." I immediately realized she had printed off pages from the posts of the online support group she read. And this stack—this stack she threw at me, was how she chose to punish me. I had never read anything about the disease before that day.

She had printed these pages back in January of that year in 2001. She had known everything—had known it all months before that night she found me drunk in my room alone. My mother had bored her wet eyes into that computer screen in the basement night after night, day after day, and never told me what in fact I found out that day.

I skimmed the first couple of pages. They were about a woman who was twenty-nine who was a caregiver for her father who had fronto-temporal dementia. The father was fifty-eight when he died. Mine, at the time of reading those papers, was fifty-one. The father in the essay had trouble with speech and then mobility. My father's speech was stunted and his math had long since left him. I decided to skip the story—I wasn't in the mood to gain strength from a stranger who was dealing with a demented father. So I turned the page and read: "The Stages of Decline." I read the introduction, the small paragraph in italic font that explained that the following stages were "the most widely accepted" in the progression of degenerative dementia. That they may be "equally applied when discussing a patient with Alzheimer's disease, Pick's disease, Multi-infarct, or other more rare forms."

I had gotten up from my bed in the middle of reading that paragraph to sit in a rolling chair beside my window. I remember because the chair kept turning back and forth on its loosened hinges and I had thought that maybe my mother had kicked it or broken it somehow the night before. I tried to steady myself by resting my feet against the window seat, resting the pages on my knees as they bent against the morning sun.

I finished the paragraph: "The time spent in any one stage varies widely, as does the overall progression of the disease. This unknown is one of the most frustrating aspects of this disease."

I imagine I may have rolled my eyes at this. I was just so utterly angry at that time—at everyone. I felt completely hopeless after having spent a summer thinking and believing things were going to get better. If things were looking up for me—then surely they would for my father. He would get better—or at least stay the same. He would stop that depression before it consumed him and I could learn to decipher his stutters.

And then I began to read the levels: "Level One . . . no memory deficit," but I knew, obviously, that it wasn't him who I read about. So I glanced over that stage and read on to "Level Two . . . forgetting names one formerly knew well . . . " and I swallowed hard. Back then—when he'd tell me about those books he got, those self-help books—he was trying to relearn words. Even then, he felt the change coming. "Level Three . . . coworkers become aware of patient's relatively low performance . . . denial becomes to be manifest," and that night when he came home from work, flustered and angered about that paragraph I had rewritten in minutes—it was a level he was ascending. "Level Four . . . concentration deficit elicited on serial subtractions . . . decreased ability to travel, handle finances . . . "; the restaurants, the tips—my mother getting anxious and annoyed watching him struggle and clear his throat, twiddling the pen between his shaking fingers. "Level Five . . . patient is unable . . . to recall . . . relevant aspects of their current lives, e.g., an address or telephone number . . . may have difficulty counting back from forty by fours or from twenty by twos . . . " How foolish of me to be annoyed at Nicole and those flashcards—those notes he kept in his wallet—"Level Six . . . will require some assistance with activities of daily living, e.g., may become incontinent . . . require assistance bathing properly . . . " and a tear slid down my face. "Level Seven . . . speech ability limited to about a half-dozen intelligible words . . . ability to sit up lost . . . ability to smile lost . . . ability to hold head up lost . . . "

And then I read again: "ability to smile lost," and a simple picture of him looking over at me, his brown eyes warm, his lasting smile, washed over my head that hung heavy as I wept.

"Ability to smile lost," and I imagined every movement upwards, every hint of a squinting eye, his lips blissfully bending upwards, an imagined crow's foot edging outwards—"Ability to smile . . . lost."

The day he'd stop smiling, forget the means to smile, the ability, the day he'd sit in solemn silence—that's the fear that bent me forward, retching drily, crying, tremors vacillating between horror and mourning for the day he would never smile—never again.

My mother didn't realize in that moment, but something in me had finally changed.

Chapter 14

My bedroom was a shambles and a mixture of time and versions of me that didn't fit together. There were the walls my sister had painted, the few keepsakes of my school years arranged on my dresser. There were taped corners of posters that had been torn from the walls. Music from my stereo played softly in the background as I swept the corner of one window seat over and sat down. Outside lay the cul-de-sac island with well-kept bushes and a tree at its center. The light of the street lamps cast their steady glow on the leaves.

In my bedroom, I only felt my most serene from that window seat, staring out into the nighttime setting of my street. Looking up, I'd see the stars shimmer with my own imaginings, alighting hope, if I had any. But mainly there was a quiet in those moments, serenaded by the songs I played. Looking outside, I could wonder what peace there was in store for my family, for me. What peace would come, and how or when? And why would peace be such an offering—when all I really wanted was my father as he was before the stages set in.

Thus, I developed the habits of a note taker, writing down every thought I had about every change I saw. Resigned to be an observer, I watched his patience now become brittle; his anger had readily become his constant companion.

On one evening, I heard him before I heard my mother. Usually, it was just the opposite. My mother's screams had varied pitch and tone that could find their way through any surface, over any distance. When she was angry, my mother's screams were thick, yet they spread evenly within a room. I would say my idea of a "yell" would better fit her version of a scream. Her yelling became so familiar that at times I just ignored them. When they weren't directed at me, I hardly heard them at all.

Except, of course, when her yelling became shrill and high. This screaming was severe and reserved for the moments when she really had no control over how to feel the anger and frustration that would overwhelm her. Watching her scream, I felt the force of all her deepest hateful moments twist around one another. Out of her mouth, it would seem as though a cyclone swept forth from her lips. These were the sounds of my mother—the sounds I heard as often as her cries.

And when she was home, which she often was, Nicole would try to calm her down.

"Mom! Please!!" She would cry. Nicole would always be the first to race towards my mother and desperately try to stop her from screaming at our father.

"Nicole—go downstairs! Please! Nicole!! Vattene!!! Vattene Nicole per l'amor di dio!" But Nicole never budged. When things became too heated, she'd finally run upstairs or run back down and slam the door to whatever room she hid within. She'd pretend to be angry, but it was despair at its most heightened level.

During the fall after our trip to Pacentro, the nerves that ran inside my father's body were triggering him to act in mysterious ways. He had already directed his frustrations at me upon returning—back when I had broken my promise and cut myself again. After that last outbreak when I had stared into his eyes for a second longer than I would have, I saw a man I never knew to be my father staring back at me. I was scared of him in that moment. More scared than I had been as a child, when he would hit my mother, or pound his head against the wall. I was more scared of him in that instant in my room than I used to be as a child, when I'd run away from him, fearing he would catch up to me and hit me harder than my mother ever could.

But I guess that comes with the territory of living in a home with Italian parents who find it more effective to slap their kids than watching them take a time out. Even my cousin Mario would try and run as fast as he could away from his father, Zio Mario. Back when we lived in New Jersey and would go to visit them. Back when I was just a year younger than Nicole was when she would try to stop the fights—I witnessed the ritual of punishment that my Zio Mario enforced on my cousin.

I had never seen him hit my cousin before that night Mario swept by me in the kitchen. He was running towards the empty dining room, trying to outrun Zio Mario. And before I really realized what was happening, I heard his screams from the other room. He was in sixth grade and so his voice was somewhere between a boy and a man.

I watched Zio Mario's shoulder blades bend and his arms fall forwards on his son's back and arms. I saw him pull his hair and Mario crying and I remember thinking, "that's just like what they do to me!" But it lasted a little longer than my own punishments or even Flavia's. And I heard my mother, "Mario—Mario, it's OK. It's OK, Mario" as she watched him helplessly.

I always knew Zio Mario was so very different from my father. He smiled less often and laughed less frequently. He didn't have that easy laugh, the throaty laugh that my father gave away so easily. His features were more rugged and his hair much more gray. And he and Zia Franca never seemed to fight.

They argued, I'm sure, but never did they have a physical fight, while my cousin Mario would watch, feeling so powerless against their anger. My sisters and I knew this side of love too well. My parent's love was turbulent, just like their tongues.

And so when Nicole tried to stop my mother from screaming at our father, my mother just turned to her and screamed even louder. "Nicole—Vattene!" My mother continued, "Giovanni! Non ce la faccio piu!" with frustration and heartbreak ignited.

It was all too much for him to stand. The shortened phrases he did manage to utter were so much more entangled within his breath. They were so much less now—so far fewer. Mainly now, they were just words. And most often, they were the words he bellowed in anger that came out as clear as the days he'd tell her, "I love you."

"Naggia Cristo!!!" I heard him bellow. I heard him shuffle his feet fast—as though he were running.

He kept yelling out a curse word—then a growl. I got up slowly from the floor and walked towards my bedroom door, ready to go downstairs and try to calm him down. I was understanding more and more that I would have to get involved. That I would have to leave the sanctity of my thoughts in my room and start showing my father that I was still his daughter—however far removed I had been, how far removed he was from his former self. I realized I needed to start battling his disease for him, as much as for me.

When I opened the door, I could see the top of his head, that bald spot beneath the hallway light marching up the stairs. And I could hear him continuing—"bitch—bitch" again and again. Then my mother from down below yelled again and he turned finally around.

"My balls!! My BALLS!! You can't—You can't!!" And hurriedly he opened his bedroom door and slammed it shut.

And downstairs, my mother would have heard the door shut as she'd return to the kitchen, back to where the argument must have started. I can see her put away the pestle and mortar, looking inside and seeing the white residue of all the pills her husband now took. He was on antipsychotic medicine, anti-anxiety, anti-depression—pills to help his anger, his emotions, his nerves that threatened to strangle him. She'd beat the medicine into dust and add it to his food to make it easier for him to take.

I can imagine her thinking, "did I give him the eye drops?" as she pushed the small box back beneath the cabinets, on the far side of the kitchen counter. He was diagnosed with glaucoma almost a year before that fall, and every night she or I, and if she were home from college, Flavia, would pry apart his nervous eyes and watch him struggle as the drops would flood his eyes.

Yes, my mother would have pushed the small box towards that small pharmacy of my father's drugs right before she'd turn to the window of the kitchen and stare out into the yard, into the changing seasons of fall into winter.

IT WAS IN winter when my mother had first stood before the window in Dr. Holtzman's waiting room, contemplating the news she had just heard—that her husband had dementia. She had, I believe, felt the draft from the cold outside reach into the core of her as she realized she would need limitless strength to undertake the journey she had in front of her.

And she had gathered enough at least to lead her down my father's twisted, disappearing journey of Alzheimer's disease. But that November in 2001, she again found herself in Dr. Holtzman's office.

She sat in front of him when he asked her point blank. I wonder what led to the question—I wonder if she confided in him, shed tears in front of him. Weeping for her husband who didn't see or seem to understand what was becoming of him. Dr. Holtzman must have asked her something, something probing, and my mother surely must have responded despondently. And so he finally asked her, "Enida, do you have any support?"

I like to imagine Dr. Holtzman had a window in his office that framed the scenes of the changing leaves and the slight wind that shook the branches of oak trees—but most likely, he didn't. Most likely, if he had a window in his office, it faced the buildings in Washington University, perhaps the skyline of the city. I can't imagine my mother looking over Dr. Holtzman's head and into the scenes of nature as she refocused her eyes on him.

Instead, I see the room encased in books and awards, perhaps a small desk lamp always lit, illuminating the sparse corners of the room where nothing save for a chair sits. I don't see a window—just the light from the lamp sharpening the contours of shadows upon my mother's face. And I hear her, feeling her caught off guard, I see her smile a bit nervously as she responds, "No—no I am doing this on my own."

"What do you mean?" Dr. Holtzman would have continued.

"No one believes me that he is sick—" she starts to tell him, and if he wore glasses at the time, Dr. Holtzman would have removed them and rubbed his eyes in disbelief as my mother told him about the simple-minded reactions of my father's brother, Zio Mario, and his sister, Zia Emma.

"They think I did this to him—that he's just depressed. His brother thinks because I am a bad wife he is this way. I tried—I tried telling them what's happening, but they don't believe me."

Zio Mario must have slammed the phone down hard after telling my mother she was a liar. And Zia Emma, one of two of my father's sisters, must have carried on with her day, perhaps just a bit angrier than she would have been had my mother not called in tears.

"I told them I think they should get tested—that it might run in families—" my mother went on, and then I remember the vision of her I imagine. I carry it with me still—the phone by her side and the sounds of her crying silently by herself.

Dr. Holtzman wrote my father's brother and sisters a letter. To each of them he detailed my father's disease and stated as drily as possible that my mother was telling the truth. To Zio Mario, the letter read:

"Dear Mr. Silvestri,   11-9-01*

I am writing this letter on behalf of Mr. John Silvestri and his wife who asked me to update several of John's relatives of his medical status. I am a Professor of Neurology at Washington University School of Medicine in St. Louis. I first saw John about two years ago. At that time, he had started to develop difficulty with language (speaking, reading, writing, and understanding words). In addition, he had begun developing trouble with problem solving. He received many tests. Following these evaluations, it was clear John was developing a dementia (trouble with thinking) due to a disease of the brain. While a definitive diagnosis of the exact cause of his dementia would require a brain biopsy, the most likely cause is Alzheimer's disease or another disease related to Alzheimer's disease called Pick's disease (fronto-temporal dementia). While these diseases are not common in people in their 40's and 50's, they do occur, and we have seen many cases. Unfortunately, there are no treatments for these diseases that prevent their progression. There are medicines which can assist with some of the problems, including behavioral problems, which he has developed. He is on some of these medicines. Over the last two years, as occurs with these diseases, John has worsened significantly. He is now moderately to severely demented. He cannot speak or understand many things. He is often quite agitated. This disease is causing this. It is likely that he now needs full-time custodialcare to take care of his daily needs (dressing, eating, going to the bathroom, etc.) His care will likely soon require services either in a nursing home or equivalent to that in a nursing home. We are trying our best to manage his problem . . . We still don't understand why some people develop these diseases and others don't. I hope this letter is of help in regards to briefly describing what has happened to John so that you are up to date.

Sincerely,

David M. Holtzman, MD

I read the letter now; a copy of one that was sent sits in our basement, in my father's old office. My mother has rehung his awards, his diplomas. Pictures of us—of Flavia, Nicole and me—adorn his small bookshelf that sits atop an old dresser in which he'd keep stashes and bundles of paper. His desk is turned now towards the wall and a list he made of his hopes and desires sits beside his small lamp. The list details plans for getting more money through stocks, plans to wear better clothes and to get a better car. He writes of plans to be happier and to read more. It is this list he wrote out on an old cardboard cutout that I think about when I read Dr. Holtzman's letter. All of the plans, however small and trivial, that were stunted and stopped.

After leaving the kitchen and turning her face away from the window, my mother would have lain again on the couch and waited until it was time for my father to take his medicine once again. I can hear her calling for me to get him to come downstairs. As I stand within his doorway to his darkened room, I can see him lying on the bed, sleeping. He seems almost peaceful.

Chapter 15

"Johnny's here!" exclaimed Linda as she opened the door and called to her son, Nicholas.

My mother grabbed a hold of my dad's arm and helped him up the small ledge before the doorway of her house. He smiled warmly as Nicholas ran towards them from the living room.

"Johnny!" Nicholas yelled as he made his way to my father. Nicholas was about three years old that morning he ran excitedly into my father's arms.

"Hi, Nicholas! Are you ready to go to the zoo with me and Johnny?" she asked him, smiling.

And I can see Nicholas beneath his thick strawberry-blond hair nod his head and smile, his nose crinkling up within the freckles on his face.

On a sunny afternoon, my mother dressed my father in blue khaki shorts and brown loafers. She put deodorant on him before putting on his red blue-striped polo tee shirt and made sure he wore his glasses. To protect his head from the sun, she had him wear a blue baseball cap with the "Illinois XXL" insignia on the front—a gift from Flavia, who was in her senior year at the University of Illinois.

During that past year or so, my father and Linda's son had been quickly becoming friends. Even as the ground grew muddy and our shoes squished in the wet grass of our neighbors' yards, our families would still make the short trip to one another's homes day or night. And just like the others, even that winter, the ground was littered with our footsteps, when the snow was not too deep. And in the coming summer, just before my parents would again fly to Italy, we'd bend the blades of the dry, yellowed grass, hearing the crunch of the branches beneath our family's willow tree. But in those seasons, the steps that seemed to change the most were of a man and a boy whose roles, it seemed, were switching.

Their steps had started melting into the same wayward gait a year or so before, back when Nicholas began to learn to walk. He crawled and grew stronger, standing between his parents and older sisters, Nathalie and Sophia. Little Nicholas took his few steps as my father began turning left instead of right in the car. My mother beside him in the passenger seat would yell at the mistake, as she still grappled with her patience in the face of the change and the new stage of his decline. I, as well, would race home and tell on him—getting more annoyed than scared at my father, who couldn't seem to drive an automatic transmission without attempting to switch gears.

And then as Nicholas would bump his knees at home, wailing and screaming, hurting from the fall that happens in learning, my own father would cry, hurting from the fall that happens from forgetting.

So on a sunny afternoon, my father sat on a stool in the bathroom, his mouth open wide while my mother silently brushed his teeth. And just behind us or in front, cattycorner in a white house, Linda stood beside little Nicholas, whose mouth barely opened wide enough for his toothbrush. It was 2001 when they both looked at themselves getting their teeth brushed in different mirrors as though synchronizing their lives in two neighboring homes.

My mother came in the early afternoon to pick up Nicholas to spend a day at the zoo. She had a lunch packed: sandwiches, bananas and juice. As my mother settled my father in the car and buckled his seat belt, Linda did the same for Nicholas before stepping back and waving goodbye.

No longer able to enjoy lunches or movies as they had just a year before, my mother had to distract my father and fill the days with more than a fifty-one-year-old man would have otherwise expected

After parking the car, my mother let out little Nicholas first and, holding his hand, made her way to the passenger's side to unlock my father's seatbelt as he shifted compulsively about in his seat. Then, she took out Nicholas's stroller and sat little Nicholas inside of it, while my mother instructed my father to stand beside her—and not in the street, where city drivers sometimes drove too fast and too close.

It was a beautiful afternoon—the sun made little Nicholas squint his eyes as he looked up to his friend Johnny. They walked hand in hand, hobbling together towards a pool of seals. Little Nicholas's red St. Louis Cardinals baseball cap sat crookedly on his head. His green tee shirt was loose-fitting and his elbows were nearly covered by the sleeves. He had a small scab on his knee below his khaki shorts. My mother checked to make sure their shoes stayed tied as they stood in the shade and watched the little boy and the middle-aged man walk alone together.

My father bent forward to get closer to his friend's height. He shuffled his feet as he tried to keep up. In pictures my mother took that afternoon, little Nicholas stands erect and confident—he seems to be leading my father. The pictures document the trepidation in Nicholas's face as he looks at his friend Johnny while the seals begin calling. They stand together in another photo: Nicholas barely reaching the top of the railing in front of a large pond. My father stands beside him, leaning against the railing and seemingly whispering to his young friend. They seemed to be babbling with each other, giggling with one another, understanding one another. In another photo, my father holds his friend in his arms, looking closely at his face, smiling as before. And Nicholas looks out before him, focusing, thinking.

Finally, they break for lunch. My mother gathers the brown paper bags from below Nicholas's stroller and gives him his sandwich and sippy cup. To my father, she too gives a sandwich and a small bottle of juice. She makes sure they start eating before she begins her own lunch.

As she peels back the skin of the bananas she brought for them, my mother stands back again and snaps a final photo.

"I didn't know who I was watching—Nicholas or Giovanni." I see her set the camera down, letting it hang on her neck by the straps as she thinks these thoughts she will later come to share with me.

MY MOTHER'S THOUGHTS certainly did become a reality sooner than we had expected. By the spring of 2002, we could never leave my father alone. He was dependent upon us for everything. Not too far from his fifty-second birthday, when the weather felt the same warmth that day at the zoo and soft breezes whispered along the sweet singing of the birds outside our home, I had fallen asleep beside my father.

I was supposed to be looking after him that afternoon as he sat in his recliner watching the stock market channel, staring at the numbers, forgetting each and every sign and symbol. At the same time, Nicholas must have been learning colors and songs on Sesame Street inside his own home. I remember trying to keep my heavy lids from falling but finally giving in to the comfort of a woven cotton blanket and a familiar warm pillow.

When I awoke, perhaps an hour or so later, the recliner by my side was empty. The television was still on; the remote control sat at the base of the chair and the recliner was still extended. I knew he had struggled to get up, having forgotten how to pull the wooden bar on the left side of the chair down. It was always easy to identify the remnants of him—the Parmesan cheese hidden in drawers, cereal spread across the table, pools of urine on the bathroom floor. But those were the times when he'd be roaming the house on his own, like a toddler with no mother.

I got up quickly, knowing he was gone, and I heard my mother screaming from upstairs, screaming that she couldn't find my father.

But the front doors were closed; his tracks were covered for the most part, and I couldn't tell which direction he had taken.

It was my first moment of real panic—the first time I felt completely helpless and powerless. The fact that I hadn't watched him, that he had escaped the safety of that living room while I slept beside him, shook me. My sisters and I would each get to know the fear that came in losing him—physically losing sight of him.

Nicole would come to share with me her most horrible memory of losing him. I remember the early evening when we sat together at the kitchen table and talked of him and the hurt from it all. I was asking her questions about this time, in 2002, when we all had nearly hit bottom.

"He just—I just, I mean, I have these memories of him, Stefania—" She cut short, stifled by her tears. She sat with her head bent downwards as I got up and stroked her back. I would never see Flavia cry in front of me, caught in the grips of a memory she'd share with me. Flavia blocks that time from me, from nearly everyone it seems. "Stef—that was my living nightmare," she tells me when I prod her. "I don't want to go back there—I *can't* go back."

Nicole, however, tries with me, though each and every time she ends in tears and I wind up with her head on my shoulder. I feel like I hurt her again and again when I ask her what she felt. But I did so only to see some of what happened through their eyes. However much they choose to give me, I use. I resolved to use only this, Nicole's most sacred and scary moment of losing her father.

"I remember coming downstairs and daddy was sitting at the table. He had poured the milk into the cereal box and was eating it. Mommy came into the kitchen and started screaming at him," here again, she began to tear up like before but resolved to continue. "And then I screamed back at her to stop—to leave him alone—"

"She was just upset, Nic; she was scared . . . "

Nicole didn't seem to hear me as she continued, "I took him upstairs with me and tried to calm him, told him it was ok. That Mommy didn't mean to get mad. He was still crying when I put him to bed and turned out the light."

I took Nicole's hand as she continued.

"And I couldn't sleep at all, Stef. I just laid down in Flavia's old bed, listening for any sounds coming from his room. And then I heard weird rustling sounds and I knew he was doing something . . . moving around. I went to his room and freaked out because he wasn't in bed but I knew he didn't go downstairs. So I went towards the bathroom, but I checked first in the closet . . . "

I know the image of what came next still lives in her, still haunts her and no way I try to retell it will ever fully paint the way the moment felt for her.

"I found him on the floor in the closet. He was sitting there, in the dark by the clothes hanging and the shoes and he was crying—crying, hysterically. I went in and took him, tucked him back in bed. I laid awake for hours, afraid that he would get up again . . . "

THAT EVENING I lost my father, I pulled open the door of my mother's car and got in. My mother's radio was on loud, and Italian music splintered my ears—I remembered cursing at her in anger as I shut it off. I pulled out of the driveway and down the street, towards that stop sign at the intersection of Cedarmill and Summer Ridge Road. There, I went with my father a week or so before during a walk we took together. My mother had told me to take him out, and I remember complaining—but quickly trying to cover up my disdain when I saw my father grow excited. We mainly walked in silence as I tried to keep our spirits high by walking on the grass, jumping up on the curb and holding his hand in mine. I led him to that intersection and then we turned left, where I was then driving. We kept going straight, right into the neighborhood across the street, where Dan lived on Easy Ridge Court. I took my father to the pond Dan and I would go to on summer days and nights when we'd smoke and drink from little miniature liquor bottles I would steal from my parents' liquor cabinet.

When my mother had caught me that night drinking alone in my room, she had poured out all the liquor and all the wine she had and threw the empty bottles in a cardboard box. She had screamed at me that I had drunk all the small liquors she and my dad had collected over the years, and I felt guilty not for the drinking, but for taking away souvenirs of their past.

The next morning, I went into the laundry room to get clothes out of the dryer and I saw the box sitting squarely in the middle of the floor. My father followed me into the laundry room and looked at me, shaking his head slightly. His eyes were large and round in that moment, and I heard him clear his voice.

"Please," he uttered softly, "Please." That's all the punishment I received from him—all the words of anger, of sadness—in the pleading from my wordless father.

THE KIDS ALONGSIDE me on their bicycles, and parents strolling by in their after supper routines, and the sun close to setting and my fears in that car were overwhelming me that day my dad ran away. Maybe he didn't see it as running away—but he did it anyway; he left.

My leg shook on the gas pedal; it struck the brakes too firmly as I jerked and sped along Baxter Road looking for him. I headed east, towards the grocery store he used to run to on weekends, on that same road Flavia used to run with him. I thought maybe he would be walking there out of habit. He used to love to go down that road on weekends. On one morning, he had yelled for me from outside and I heard him from the kitchen. "Stefania! Come here!"

I walked quickly towards the garage door in the laundry room, and when I opened it I saw him standing there, sweating, glowing and giddy. He motioned for me to follow him out into the garage. And when I did, he grabbed my hand and led me to the driveway.

"I was running and I just saw it in the grass—"

And below us on the cement sat a medium-sized box turtle, with one leg shriveled and small. I look up at my father as I laughed, "A turtle!! Thank you daddy!!!"

"I was running down the street, holding this turtle in one hand and people were looking at me wondering what I was doing," he said as he picked up the nervous turtle as it quickly shrank inside its shell.

That evening, just an hour or so after having sectioned off a small area of grass with logs that would act as my new pet's home, I went out to check on it. As I looked down, I was shocked at what I saw—the home I had made was empty—my turtle had run away. With only three legs, it still had managed to disappear in just a couple of hours left on its own.

I DROVE AND drove and it seemed like I had driven much too far for my demented father to have traveled in such a short time. Sweat poured from my face and from under my arms. I smelled of hot, sickening discomfort, and then I saw him.

He was stumbling, grumbling—hunched over, his arms at his side. He seemed to be walking unnaturally stiff and bent forwards. I rolled down the window, swerved a bit and yelled to him. I beeped at him to startle him, to slow him down. But he kept walking.

"Daddy!" I yelled, "Stop! What's the matter with you?!" I pulled into a driveway to cut his path on the sidewalk and his eyes were furrowed and dark and he shook his head as cars whizzed by us. "Get in the car, dad. Come on," I told him, and he shook his head.

"Vattene! Naggia dio, lasciami!" he screamed at me, telling me to go, and I stood still, surprised at the fluidity in his speech. I remembered being blown away at his heated anger and hearing his voice he hid away for so many years since he'd been sick. My father did seem to hold onto Italian curse words the longest—they seemed to be his shell when all else failed.

"Please daddy, please, let's go home."

After I finally talked him into getting back inside the car, I locked the doors. I remained silent like him as we turned to drive down Baxter once more.

The next day, my mother told me to pick up childproof doorknob covers at Wal-Mart. Since I worked there, I could get a discount and I felt useful, in a way, to be able to save her a bit of money.

The infant department stood next to the shoe department where

I worked. I hated that job—hated organizing and reorganizing the shoes after customers would leave them scattered in the aisles. I liked my managers, the two blond and heavyset women in their forties. They respected me and seemed to like me. I guess it's because I mainly kept to myself and worked without talking. I learned to go to work with the intention of working only. My mother used to remind me back when I worked at the movie theatre, "Stefania, you go to work to *work*, not make friends." And as a tribute to her, I tried my best to do just that at Wal-Mart. Plus, the people my age seemed distracted in their high schools and their crushes. Whereas they would have friends and relatives come and walk through their departments, chatting in the aisles, my father would show up randomly side-by-side with my mother, or at times with Flavia and Nicole. Once, Flavia jokingly dropped some shoes on the ground and my father glared at her angrily. "I'm just joking, dad! God!" she exclaimed as she quickly picked them up. "It's OK dad," I told him, smiling to show him I meant it.

Flavia would remain stunned at our father's quick anger—and Nicole would laugh at both the humor in it, and the awkwardness. Before they'd turn to leave, I'd imagine the look of pride that would wash across his furrowed brow. And I'd stand watching them leave together, wishing I could join them—wishing maybe even more that I could throw each and every shoe on the ground on my way out.

I stood nervously in the infant department with a red basket hanging from my limp, shaking arm. There were so many different types of cupboard locks, fancy medicine bottle lids, and two different kinds of doorknob covers.

I stood still, biting the inside of my bottom lip, picking my fingernails bare. Finally, I grabbed one of the doorknob covers I thought looked secure. Should I get two? Four? I pictured all of the doors in our house—the door to the garage—that would be important. The front door—of course. The back door—what if he found a way to open the basement door and get confused by the stairs? I bought enough for every door in the house.

After loading my basket, I walked silently towards the cashiers.

A few days later, friends asked me what those covers were for—I told them all they were to keep the doorknobs clean. "They were getting rusty," I said. The truth I only told to Dan—he responded with just enough pity and concern, just like I knew he would.

My dad's last birthday at home was on March 20, 2002. He turned fifty-two that day. My mother had made pasta, feeding it to him after cutting it up in small pieces. Nicole and I cleaned up the table as our mother was finishing up with him—she had already finished eating, sitting down before any of us so that she could devote more time to feeding her husband. She had to be careful not to feed him too much too fast, as she had a habit not only of walking fast, but of eating fast as well.

When he was done eating, we brought out a chocolate cake with a lit candle in the center. He smiled—I remember it well. And then he slowly puckered his lips and set them tenderly on my mother's cheek as Nicole took a picture with her Izone camera. It was her favorite toy at the time—a small, rectangular camera that would develop instant pictures on inch-by-inch film. In the living room, behind the television and on top of a bookshelf, pictures from my father's birthday lie displayed in a multiple-picture frame. The one of my father's kiss is placed above the rest, and I imagine it sometimes as being the last kiss he ever gave his wife freely—in a rare moment of near total lucidity.

Chapter 16

Flavia called me on the phone the week before my 18th birthday, which was just a couple weeks ahead of my father's 52nd that March of 2002—"Stef, do you want to come up and visit? I think you'd have a lot of fun up here. It'll be nice and it'll give you a chance to get away." She spoke affectionately as she tried to sway me to come and see her. I stood in front of the pantry, trying to decide what to eat for breakfast as well as trying to decipher if she spoke in earnest when she told me she wanted me there. It hadn't been that long since my mother had called, screaming into the phone that I had been drinking alone in my bedroom. I didn't want Flavia to feel forced to have me. She had enough to worry about and I was sick and tired of having to be her priority.

"Alright, Fla. I'll come."

I didn't know it then, but just a couple of months before, my mother had started looking at nursing homes with a friend. And in the midst of my mother's planning for the future she seems not to have overlooked even her daughters. "Flavia, she's always in her room—I don't know if it's Giuseppe or your father—but I need your help," I can see her tell Flavia over the phone, as my imagination looms over her tense conversation in the kitchen. I never did know if she had told her or not; simply that my family was trying to keep itself intact is all I do know for certain.

The few days I spent with Flavia were relaxing, and I remember I was happy. We stayed in her apartment in the afternoons when we didn't go out for lunch or meet a friend of hers at a bar she would frequent. "Stef—I used to come here after the basketball team would play. A bunch of us would come and I think I even got kicked out once—"

"What!?" I asked her, nearly choking on the soda I was slurping.

"It wasn't a big deal—everyone knew me; it was so much fun," she told me as we sat beneath a hanging lamp in a booth, surrounded by television screens and the thick scent of beer and college. Later, she told me that was the same bar a guy had casually told her she resembled a Fraggle from a favorite childhood television of ours, *Fraggle Rock*. Even that story had us erupting in laughs—both of us filling our corner of the restaurant in seal-like laughter, sounding more like we were gasping for breath than taking a break from ourselves for a moment in hysterics.

Flavia had a boyfriend at the time named Mike. He and I stayed in her apartment one night while she went to the library to study for a final.

"So you like this movie?" he asked me as he lay opposite me on Flavia's couch. We had gone to the video store to rent a movie and I had chosen *The Crow*.

"Yeah," I told him. I had known I would be watching a movie with him while Flavia studied, so I purposefully chose a film that may have helped to validate my position as the depressed younger sister. It certainly would help me relax despondently on the couch, at least, which is what I ultimately wanted to do. As much as I seemed to hate my depression, I needed it—*craved* it, rather.

I knew Mike was trying to be kind and trying to find some common ground with me. And I was trying, too—trying to keep my distance from this boy who seemed too far removed from the life I wanted desperately to escape. I was also spiteful that he was even there. I was jealous that Flavia was in college—that she was away from home and free to do what she wanted. I was jealous she had this boy who loved her when the boy who loved me had abandoned me and left me hurting more than I had before I met him.

I kept a shroud upon me heavily because I believed it was how I was meant to be. I wasn't meant to be happy—wasn't meant to be loved, and I surely didn't deserve to be.

A WOMAN NAMED Marianne who lived in our neighborhood accompanied my mother to the nursing homes. Around that time, Nicole was good friends with her daughters and would often be found playing at her house after school. I would honk the horn of the Volvo station wagon as I waited for her outside. But she hardly ever heard the call. As I would walk up the stone pathway towards their front door, an old woman would often answer. She was their grandmother—with white hair, large, round glasses, and lips so frail and worn. Years later, she would move to another house belonging to one of her children—succumbing to the effects of dementia herself.

And it seems that my mother was faced with her most trying times always when the weather was cold, when the winter shrunk the promises of starting over and the new beginnings often found in spring. She would have had her tennis shoes on, a large dark coat and perhaps something else she wore to keep out the fear that day she stepped inside Marianne's car.

THAT SAME MORNING must have been a school day, though if it were I doubt my father was at home alone. If it were a school day, I most assuredly would have been in the Volvo, dropping off Dan at school. He had found another problem with his car, had gotten into an accident again, or the car must have broken down again. "I don't know why they keep giving me old cars! Of course they're going to break!" he'd say and I would invariably agree with him. But only because I loved him. Inside, I would wonder why, really—I mean, *how* can you go through cars as fast as cigarettes? Because by that time, Dan was a full-fledged smoker. He smoked and smoked, more than even I seemed to smoke, and I had at least a couple of years ahead of him.

"So what—your eyes don't hurt anymore?" I asked him as he inhaled deeply from his cigarette and blew the smoke in my face. "Oh yeah?" I continued, in a whiny and nasally voice.

He smiled and laughed, tilted his head back and then looked again at me. I sort of felt a little bad seeing him smoke now almost crazily.

But he was eighteen now and my glove compartment overflowed with Camel Lights now that Dan—day or night—could go and buy them for me whenever I needed them.

"Well, my parents smoked for twenty-five years and now my dad runs marathons," he'd tell me, defiantly. As much as he was annoyed with me back when he didn't smoke, Dan was now completely taken with smoking and with defending it with all he had. "I mean, you've seen how good-looking my mom is—her face isn't *gray*."

He knew what I wanted to hear—I had an obsession with thinking smoking was turning my face gray. But really, the only parts of my face that were gray were the bags beneath my eyes that came mainly from oversleeping, not sleeping, and simply not feeling at all well.

"Dan, I'm just going to drop you off. I feel like shit again today—" I told him as we neared the high school.

"Oh yeah?" He asked me in that same nasally and whiny voice.

"Yeah—I'm sorry. I just need to drive. I can't stand it anymore. I can't breathe—" I told him as I drove up to the front of the school like my father used to do back when he remembered how.

"You sure? Come on—I'll go to Denny's with you. I'll buy," he said.

"No—no I'm just gonna go," and I recall I often teared up at these points. If not in front of Dan, then as I drove away from him. I didn't like always feeling separate from him or from any of the students I saw walking sleepily up to school. Whoever they were or however they felt inside—I was convinced I was separate from them in every way. That my suffering could never compare to theirs was my conviction as I drove away from Dan and all the rest of the days I'd skip school and find myself driving aimlessly around West County.

I WONDER IF my mother printed lists of nursing homes off the Internet—or if she hand-wrote them on paper she'd find in our drawers in the kitchen. The paper she would have found would have that irksome smile from a realtor and how ironic would it have been if

Seth Neally stared up on the notepad from which she wrote. He sold us our house when we had moved in nearly eight years before. And that morning, my mother was on her way, staking out new homes where only my father would then reside.

So it was that around the same time I was driving away from school, from Dan who must have met up with friends at the door and laughed his way to his locker, my mother walked up the stairs to a nursing home with Marianne. The doors, I'm sure, were automatic and slid easily apart as she entered in the homely waiting areas where sat a door attendant who would have called for the director to meet with the two women who stood awkwardly waiting. The director would have met them both near the attendant's desk, and, while shaking the director's hand, my mother would have introduced herself: "I am Enida—my husband John has Alzheimer's disease."

Did the director smile, shocked, at the woman in her late forties speaking of her husband in his early fifties? I hear the clicks of the director's heels as she led the two women to the Alzheimer's Unit that must have been separated from the rest. As the director opened the door, I imagine Flavia turning the pages of her book back in Illinois, studying for an exam she would have the next day. Nicole, I'm sure, was laughing with her friends in front of her first locker in sixth grade—her round glasses now replaced by a pair of brown, rectangular frames that matched her eldest sister's.

And my father—I can see him pacing the house, back and forth, sitting, standing, feeling lost and empty. But he, again, would not have been home alone—one of us would have been there with him. So it surely must have been a weekend when my mother first visited a nursing home. Of that first visit—she remembers the horror she felt, clearly as though she dreamed it the night before, "it was terrible and scary . . . some smelled so bad . . . and one I liked was very expensive . . . the one I thought was okay was Bethesda . . . "

Bethesda would become a name we would all know well not too far from then—but upon first seeing it, upon first seeing the Alzheimer's ward, my mother says, "The door locked behind me and people were sitting in recliners, chairs, holding dolls and trying to get me to let them out. I left crying."

"The regular?" Dan asked Laura, the woman with the drawn-in eyebrows. We had learned her name after Dan had started talking to the baristas. Apparently, they had all had a crush on Dan—calling him, "beautiful eyes," and of course, he was the first between us who got his regular.

Dan and I began going to The Grind with another friend of ours, Jessie. She was a friend of Dan's from drama class and she and I started to become close as she started spending more time with Dan. She was a born-again Christian, a music lover—especially of hard rock. She gave Dan and me the right amount of optimism and joy with her easy laugh. Her dimples in her cheeks were addictive to watch as was her style—with her short, often dyed red hair and her bell-bottomed jeans. Jessie was a mixture of personalities and tastes, but her kindness and her spirituality made her completely unlike anyone Dan and I had ever known.

"You sure you don't want to go with us to the concert tomorrow?" she asked me one night as Dan stood by the counter, chatting with his new fan club.

"Oh, Jess. I can't. You know I have to be home by 11:30—and especially now that my mom is crazy and my dad is even worse," I told her, taking a deep breath and lifting an eyebrow at "worse."

"Yeah, I know—I'm really sorry about what you are going through, Stefania. I can't imagine—" she started.

Dan lit his cigarette before sitting down with us. "So I'm going to Darren's tonight I think. He's having some of his lesbians over too—" Dan said, "I met a couple of them last weekend. They seem nice."

"Dan—is this the guy you started dating a couple of weeks ago?" Jessie asked, as she took a sip of her coffee. Her rings on her fingers hit against the white mug as the corners of her eyes creased.

"Yeah—you remember him, right Stefania? He was tall, had brown hair—you claimed he was balding—" Dan said, smirking as he looked over at me sitting to his side. I was fiddling with a lighter with the green sleeves of Dan's oversized sweatshirt he had lent me nearly covering my hands. My black nails scratched the sides of the orange-and-yellow Bic that Dan and I had purchased together on one of our drives. We always seemed to lose a lighter, or need a quick pick-me-up of Dr. Pepper on afternoons we'd drive together.

"Stefania—ugh, see Jess? She's not even listening—" Dan said. He was mainly making a point to Jessie rather than showing me his disdain. They both were well aware that my mind was almost always filled to excess.

"Dan—don't piss me off. You know all the shit I have to think about?" I didn't always try my best with him. "And he is balding—not to mention thirty years older than you."

"Uh, try eight." Dan said, as he put his hand to his chest, over-exaggerating his correction.

"OK Dan—Stefania, what did your mom say when you told her Dan asked you to the prom over the intercom at school?" Jessie asked.

"Oh my god—she thought it was hilarious—Dan did you really call her to get the translation?" I asked him, suddenly perking up.

"Yeah—she said it was 'vuoi venire al ballo con me' so I just tried to think of rhyming words to go with it—" he said. "She didn't understand what I meant by intercom though."

"She probably thought you meant the same thing Marc used last year when he asked me. Remember? That handheld loudspeaker when he picked me up?" Jessie started laughing as she remembered. Her laughter came in waves as Dan joined in too. Dan's laugh was heavier and he opened his mouth wider when he laughed than when he spoke. Together, he and Jessie got the best of me as I begrudgingly laughed along with them.

"Yeah—I told him how funny I thought that would be—he went to three stores looking for one!" I said. Just last year, Marc had picked me up for school in his mother's Jeep. Like Dan, Marc knew how to make me forget. I could be myself and let myself slip the farthest without fear or reserve. Marc and I liked and loved to laugh with one another. With Marc, I could make jokes about anything and he would find it amusing. We would sing together—but unlike singing with Dan, Marc was content to merely "talk loudly" in a monotone voice. He looked a lot like Dan, except his eyebrows were much thicker. Dan flitted about as a gymnast when he was a small boy—while Marc's childhood weight kept him grounded in front of the television. Marc was loyal and centered, while Dan's emotional extremes and humor matched me more in the end.

Back on my sixteenth birthday, it was Marc who I called to pick me up and take me away from my house. It was Marc who I ran to frantically as my mother and father chased me. I had my hand on Marc's car door handle as my mother pulled my hair towards her and my father grabbed my arms. I had disobeyed them in some way, was punished and grounded. But I wanted desperately to run away. It was not too far from the time I spat in my father's face. He was trying to pull me off my mother's bed as I screamed at him, "I hate you." I followed that with the act I had seen in countless movies—though the regret I felt was so different than what I thought I would feel: victorious, audacious. Instead, what I remember most from that moment is the way he winced when he saw me do it and then paused for a second as he stared into my guiltless face.

Not too long before graduation, Dan came to my house to pick me up for our senior prom. I had borrowed Linda's black and beaded dress. I didn't want to buy a new one and my mother was already too stressed with my father. They had all left to visit Flavia, who was graduating from college that same weekend. I chose to stay and be with Dan rather than go—and I do believe it was the better choice. Nicole would tell me how my mother had screamed at my father, who sat beside her in the passenger seat. He would try and unlock the door, telling her, "Let's go." Nicole remembers clearly the tension that filled those three hours as his anxieties clashed with my mother.

During the graduation, they sat on wooden auditorium benches. My father kept wanting to stand or get up and leave. And my mother—she would grab his arm and tell him, "Giovanni—please sit down. Flavia is graduating. Look—look and see Flavia. She's graduating college, Giovanni."

I don't know too much about that day because Flavia and I never spoke in detail about it. Again, she chooses to lock it inside her and I am left with the perhapses of what it must have been like that afternoon. I see a picture in my mind of a photograph my mother took after the ceremony. Flavia stands beside her father while holding her diploma. His hands are behind his back and he's smiling. He actually looks proud standing beside his eldest daughter, who seems taller than he in that moment. Nicole stands on the other side of him, her short hair a bit askew from the wind, her feet tilted towards them both. She's smiling from everything inside of her. Ever my version of joy, Nicole's smile is the anchor to every fleeting worry or care. Flavia's smile at that moment nearly matches Nicole's—in that it's pure, it's sincere. Flavia's smile seems to have hidden any fear and grief she must have felt knowing she would soon be moving home once again.

THAT NIGHT AT prom, Dan and I snuck out to sit on a bench outside the hotel where prom was held and smoked cigarettes and talked about the finality that seemed to settle all around us that evening.

"Well, Stefania, this is it. This is our senior prom," he said as I stooped over to take off my dress shoes and swing them gently beneath me.

"Yup. This is it—wish we had something to drink," I said, dissatisfied with the supposedly momentous evening.

"Wish you didn't tell me I was so sweaty—" Dan started to say as I looked over at him and rolled my eyes.

After the dance, Dan, Jessie and I and a few others went to The Grind just down the street. We sat among friends at a table outside, enjoying the evening before we were to leave and go to a party of which I have no recollection. I only recall the pleasure I felt in the moments we shared at The Grind. I hear as though it were through water the sounds of cackling and snorting—the jokes we made and the plans we shared. I remember the warm evening against my bare arms, the smells of coffee and cigarettes—the image of myself picking the bobby pins out of my hair as it gently falls against my back.

My high school graduation was not too far after Flavia's from college, but the picture I keep of that day is much different. I recall standing alphabetically with my peers in the auditorium for the ceremony. And not too far from my left sat Nicole, my mother and my father in the front row on folding chairs. My mother had told me to request handicapped seating and in my request, I had had to mention my father's disability of "Alzheimer's disease."

I tried to spot the look of wonderment in my friends' eyes—those besides Dan and Jessie. I wanted them to see my father sitting in the front row, his eyes looking tired and dark, his belly protruding over his jeans, his continence challenged.

Still angry and still spiteful, I wanted recognition beyond mere pity. I was graduating high school and my father looked as though he couldn't have cared less. I wondered if he even knew what was happening. Nicole sat dutifully as always with her headphones on as she and my mother watched me walk up on the stage and shake the hand of my principals. When I shook the hand of Ms. Harlen, who just two years before had watched me cry beside my parents during my meeting with the school board after I had been caught smoking marijuana, she smiled into my eyes warmly. It felt as though I was finishing up a troubled era of skipping classes and missing Giuseppe and that I could finally leave all of that behind as I began my new life as a college-bound graduate.

I looked at my mother as I walked by in front of her. She was calling my name and cheering me on as my father sat quietly beside her. But in my mind, I had heard him cheering along with my mother.

AFTER MY GRADUATION, Flavia moved home. She was going to begin working full-time for Boeing and help take care of my father. Unfortunately, that July my father ran away again.

I was working more than ever at Wal-Mart not too long after tossing my cap into the air and exhaling deeply for what I thought would be closure for a few of the worst years of my life. My parents had made plans to go alone to Italy in August and so the majority of that early summer was spent in anticipation of their departure.

That morning in July when he ran away again, my father awoke early, agitated and stressed. It had become his pattern to awake suddenly and roam the house with worry. Since my sister had moved back home, my mother was free to leave the house when she felt herself near a breaking point—though she often let herself erupt nonetheless. Yet that day, she had decided to go to the mall to unwind and do some shopping for their trip.

Leaving my father with Flavia, she drove the ten minutes it took to arrive at the Chesterfield Mall.

And what I know now are only the pieces left from my mother's memory.

That morning in July, my sister had gone upstairs, and in that time the agitated man had left the house. Before my mother reached our cul-de-sac, she came across Marianne driving by and coming to a stop. "Enida—your husband is gone. We're all out looking for him," Marianne told her as my mother quickly panicked. Outside our home, she found Flavia standing among neighbors and friends, all of whom were on the search for my father.

"Naggia Cristo! Flavia! I told you to watch him!" She yelled, as Flavia cried the hardest she had in months.

"I was only upstairs for a little bit—I know—I know I shouldn't have," she tried to explain as my mother joined the search with the neighbors.

They were all standing there outside in groups, talking amongst one another, worrying and praying. Linda was there and even neighbors we never really talked to much before. And the police came by shortly after my mother had frantically called 911. "My husband is missing—he's sick," she must have told them and then began the twisted tale of his illness.

So as they all heard the sirens streaming across Baxter Road, the neighbors, my mother and sister stood in disbelief as two police cars pulled up to the house. They were frantic, I'm sure, but a part of them was thankful knowing they were not alone anymore. It seemed we had our entire neighborhood on our side, in search of my father, the agitated man with dementia.

By law, my mother said, the police had to check our home, do a search of the premises. They must have waited outside—Flavia still crying and my mother still panicking. When the police scoured each floor, each room where my father wandered day after day, they found nothing. They sat my mother down and got a description of what he was wearing—jeans and a white tee shirt. She showed them pictures of him—a man in his early fifties, black hair with specks of gray, black mustache, medium build. They also gathered from my mother that he had Alzheimer's disease and he had been, lately, very fussy and easily angered. He would seem disoriented, perhaps even appear like he was "on drugs"—but, she said, "he's just sick and I need him back home. It's getting late and it's so hot outside. Please—please find him."

It would take two hours to find my father that day he ran away the second time. After my mother had sat down with police in her home, seven were dispatched to go find him. Had they not found him within a half hour of their search, they would have sent for a helicopter. It was getting dark outside and the chances of finding him at night would have made the search even harder.

But then, a police officer *did* find my father. He was near the Chesterfield Mall when they drove up to him, noticing first, perhaps, his white shirt clinging to his sweaty back.

When they dropped him off at home, he was so calm. He "seemed fine, like it didn't even faze him," my mother would tell me. "He got out and I took him to the living room and he sat on his chair and just watched TV." How strange must it have been for the police that day and everyone involved—searching for a middle-aged man, finding him and then taking him home again to a wife who claimed he had dementia. How very strange indeed to watch him walk slowly into the house and take up the rest of the evening as though nothing out of the ordinary had even happened.

And still, she doesn't know how he did it—how he managed to cross the busy intersection of Baxter Road and Clarkson Road. My mother still doesn't understand how he managed to walk that far to the mall when he could scarcely find his footing to the bathroom or his bedroom. Maybe, she wonders, he was looking for *her*. She had gone to the mall that day and had even told him so. Maybe my father was looking for his wife, wanting to join her, hold her hand in his, and accompany her on a nighttime stroll back home.

Chapter 17

Driving among the towns of Abruzzo that speckled the surrounding mountains and valleys, I began to feel anxious. I didn't know how much longer we had, except that we were closer now and that my time with my father was getting shorter. I looked out the window to my right, imagining passing over Nicole's sleeping eyes as she undoubtedly must have been asleep beside Flavia, who drove behind us in angst. Zio Marco was known for driving wildly, as though all of the words he never uttered beside my mother, who bemoaned her loss behind petty talk and conversation, overcame him as he pressed further down on the accelerator. Flavia's will to stay in line with her uncle may have faltered as she saw the point of risking her safety and Nicole's as meaningless. She, I can plainly almost see in detail, would have released her grip on the wheel, would have released her foot's pressure against the accelerator—would have glanced quickly at Nicole just as I seemed to do then. And she would have known in an instant what mattered more than running away.

In the midst of this battle of driving, I dreaded seeing the castle in Pacentro rise ahead of us, just beyond the bend of the road. I felt pain knowing I would never be this close to my father again. It was that same feeling I would get saying goodbye to him before getting up and leaving, turning my head back to catch a glimpse of him, hoping he had understood my goodbye.

Yet how many times had I driven through this area and mistook Pacentro for another town that lay ahead of us in the distance? Since I was a child I had seen these same towns from windows of cars and trains and moments in time that have woven together in the story of us, in the essence of who we had become. Nicole would awaken soon, no doubt and be the first to squeal in excitement, "We're almost there—we're almost there!" Maybe my mother's own thoughts would harmonize alongside her daughter's, in octaves much lower, "Siamo qui—finalmente—siamo arrivati," in more of a sigh of relief.

By then we had driven a couple of hours in Zio Marco's speeding car and would shortly be approaching the small road that would lead to the intersection of busy roads that lead to Pacentro.

But there was time left still—time for me to rest, still, with my foot against his urn. My thoughts traced the outlines of the clouds whispering outside our car, the mountains humming along with the undulating pulses of our heartbeats. I had known this was coming—I knew it from the moment I sat down beside him and withstood the panic and nausea of keeping my feet away from his urn. To finally feel free enough to touch it—to know I would soon lose it—reminds me of the times, usually at night, when I would come so close to thinking I had lost that man for good.

I sat alone in the dining room not too long before he and my mother traveled to Italy together for the last time.

My mother was out, I'm sure to the mall to get away. I had put my father to bed, tucked him in and turned out the lamp that sat at his bedside. He never really used to read before bed—that was more my mother's style. And I would hear him complain to her—"Come on—come on, turn the light off"—from their open doorway in my room.

I sat on the dining room floor that evening in the dark with my legs bent against my chest; I tried hard to just sit and not be tempted to hurt myself in order to manage that pain I had in me. And as I sat there, I imagined I heard him. So clearly I heard him call for me, "Stefania!" It was the same tone he'd use when wanting to get my attention, when he wanted me to look at something with him—to go outside and meet him, or run downstairs and see him. It was that voice I heard, and in a moment I didn't breathe. I didn't move a muscle until I suddenly ran as fast as I could up the stairs and heard only his snoring from that open doorway to his bedroom.

I stood beside the door and contemplated leaving, going back down the stairs and pretending my moment of hysteria had never happened. Instead, I crept inside and lay beside him. My mother's side didn't sink like his did—his had a permanent sink hole in the center shaped like him, and I imagine it'd be the same outline of his body if he lay down upon the snow.

"Dad? Daddy?" I whispered so as not to wake him, "Daddy—I love you," and I cried harder than I meant to as I uttered those words. I shook the bed with my trembling, silent cries and then I woke.

"Stefa? Are you okay?" He asked me clearly. He never spoke at that point, only grunted, perhaps pointed, maybe even laughed. But he never spoke—not like that moment. It made me smile. I realized I still had him, however short a time I had left and however faraway he seemed—I still had him.

AND I WONDER where were my sisters in that moment when I realized we were near Pacentro? Were they still driving with their windows down? Were the cool, soft breezes from the Adriatic Sea seemingly embracing them, bracing them? I think Flavia needed that time alone to drive beside Nicole, who depended on Flavia's strength to get her through the drive.

Like Nicole, I depended on Flavia as well.

"Fla—what should I major in? English? Should I just put that down for now?" I asked her as she drove me to the university I would attend that fall for orientation. I had forms I had yet to complete for registration on my lap. Choosing my major seemed like it could wait until the drive.

"Stef—what is wrong with you? You're asking me *now* what you should major in? Wow, Stef," she said as she looked at me incredulously.

Just a couple of months afterwards, Flavia would again drive me when I moved to college. She had packed up the car that morning with my boxes of stuff I had prepared for my dorm room. She had filled the gas tank and checked the maps again. She even hired my friend Marc to cut the lawn the morning we left and as we drove out of the parking lot, I yelled to him, "Bye, Marc! I'm going to college! See ya!"

And during that drive to college, my mother and father in Pacentro were most likely sitting down to dinner at my father's cousin Angiolina's house. She was the young girl of my father's memories who ran in the streets alongside him near their homes, drinking the icy water from the spigots at the end of their street, running in tattered clothes, no doubt, and rough and scabbed knees. Angiolina grew to be a homely woman, living with her husband and daughter and sick mother, Nonna Conncetta's younger sister. No doubt, my mother held a fork of pasta up to my father's eager lips as my sister looked at me and said, "Stef, don't worry. I'll help you move everything in—and after we can get lunch—OK?"

THAT SUMMER OF 2002, my mother had decided to take my father to Italy, back to Pacentro for what she already knew was to be his last time ever going. Dr. Holtzman had warned her about the trip, telling her it would be better if she'd stay home, that the journey would be too much for either of them.

My mother's determination is relentless, so she bought those tickets for August and prepared herself for what she knew would be hard—but turned out to be harder than expected.

So on an August morning, I said goodbye to both of them and went to work at Wal-Mart. I would spend the majority of my time in the backroom on the hidden desk nearer the back stock of shoes and write poetry about losing my father, about having lost Giuseppe. I would write of a pain that felt immense, and I would come to feel close to metaphors of sadness in the same way that I would soon feel a closeness with love, familial love of a kind I never knew could be healing.

And my parents went to the airport en route to Rome.

Flavia had moved back home from college during the summer, so I imagine while I scribbled away in the backroom of Wal-Mart, she dutifully packed up the car and drove my irritated mother and agitated father to the airport. Nicole, had she gone along? Or did they tell her there was no room for her? My sick father needed all the attention and my mother needed space—as much as she could gather. Nicole was twelve—she had her bangs, though they were growing out, and I imagine her braces made her feel a little more awkward than older. I wonder if she awoke that day to an empty house, poured herself some milk, fixed herself a bowl of cereal and watched *Rugrats* on the television, even though she surely must have been too old for that show.

MY MOTHER SAYS the plane ride was the worst part. He never wanted to sit down. He was like a topsy-turvy toddler who just wants to stand, just wants to yell, just wants to do anything but sit still. My father would murmur, "Let's go," while my mother would exclaim, "Sit down! Please! We're going to Pacentro! Giovanni, siediti. Siediti, Giovan—" perhaps even blushing at the stares of the passengers surrounding her.

Except my mother doesn't blush. She confronts. Had there been a complaint, she would have fought back. She is a fighter and protector—a maintainer of the dignity that my father was seemingly losing each and every day.

I stared at my empty dorm room—half empty really; my roommate had already moved in. Her name was Ashley and she was a sorority girl. I looked around at her color-coordinated trinkets, her colorful stationery and stuffed animals and the sentiments of frivolity that I was far from understanding.

"Oh my god, Fla. I'm living with Marcia Brady." Ashley's photographs decorated her desk, her long, wavy hair, majestic eyes and winning grin captivated even me for a second before I hid it behind sarcasm and disdain.

"Alright—alright, it's OK, Stefania. Maybe she's nice. . . . Um, here, do you want me to set up?" But before I even spoke, she was already arranging my desk to fit my computer, adjusting Ashley's nightstand in order to make room for my fan. Ashley had called bottom bunk so I was stuck with the top. I watched as Flavia climbed up to my bed and started setting the sheets on, folding the corners in, making my bed look comfortable.

At one point, I remember her falling off the bed and us laughing. I loved Flavia more than I had known before. I watched her try to ease my anxiety as I stood there in horror not just because of my new Brady Bunch roommate, but because of the size of the room, of not knowing how to move in, and the fact that I was now on my own. Alone.

MY MOTHER SAYS she never felt so alone as that summer month in Pacentro. She never felt so distant as she did on those hot days, with the beads of sweat dropping down her brow and his.

Sitting on the old couch set against the wall in Angiolina's living room—facing the small, round wooden table adorned with a table mat to protect the finish—my father sat with empty eyes. He never did give much eye contact anymore. Sure enough, in a moment, those still eyes would turn into agitated eyes—and then, without warning or pause, panicked eyes. My mother would see the change and nod to Angiolina, who could see her from the slight doorway to the kitchen. My mother would look at her husband again, maybe tell him, "Siediti, Giovan—Angiolina sta preparando la cena," so that his nerves would calm at the mention of dinner.

And perhaps the only one in the room who may have glanced at my father during those hours in his cousin's apartment was his aunt. She sat slackened in her comfy chair, her mouth open, her white hair wispy and deadened. She hardly spoke a word but penetrated the quiet moments between stories and laughter of the guests in her daughter's home with her sickly presence. She was around the age of eighty or more and suffering spells of dementia. I like to think that in the presence of conversation and looks and murmurs that may have passed over my father, he and his aunt understood each other's language and felt each other's presence a bit more acutely, and, in a way, more warmly, then the steam rising from the bowl of pasta and meatballs and sausage that Angiolina would lay heavily before her guests.

FLAVIA LEFT ME later that afternoon after hugging me tightly. I waited for her to reverse out of the parking spot before I walked towards the park—Peace Park—that lay just on the other side of the street from my dorm. I approached a bench where I would come to spend late nights chain smoking and weeping during moments I would find myself completely lost and mournful for a time in life when I didn't have my scars—when cutting meant falling on the cement steps near the sidewalk to Nonna Concetta's home. A time when love was something gentle and guilt was just an excuse for getting out of trouble.

So in the midst of my newfound freedom, I befriended a man in my dorm who could buy me alcohol. He had been in the military, or was about to be. I didn't care much about him except that he was older than the rest of us who lived in the dorm. He had a zebra-printed futon he'd ask me to sit on when I'd enter his room with my hand filled with cash.

"Um, maybe just a pint? Or whatever you can buy with a twenty—" I'd tell him, "Jack Daniels." Still, in the grimmest of times, Jack Daniels was my beverage of choice. Before he could start in on the "you're beautiful"s, and the "why don't you sit right here on my futon"s I'd be out of there and up again in my room. Or regrettably, I'd leave with him and we'd walk down the gray stone stairs of the dorm, bypassing smokers and the butts I had aided in amassing—and I'd wait for him in the parking lot. I'd like to say I never did go in the car with him and drive to the liquor store, never sat beside him and watched my reflection in the mirror, thinking about how false I seemed and felt, pretending I was so tough behind my grungy facade I had worn since middle school.

But then I'd hear the car door slam and see myself thanking him again with the smell of his car still around me as I made my way up to my room. I'd throw the bottle in a drawer and hide it behind old shirts that all looked the same and think for a second what would happen if I had a search go on in my room—would they tell my family? Would my mother find out? Did I pause a second longer and imagine the two of them in the moment before I shut the drawer and hear the bottle roll sideways?

But before I'd have a moment to dwell too much on them, a friend would have knocked on my door—one in particular who would become my closest friend that year.

"Hi, Stefania. Whatcha doin? I brought you a book I thought you might like . . . " she told me that first night of our friendship. I let her in, a woman of nineteen with dark, shoulder-length brown hair and black-framed glasses. She was full-figured with curves I'm sure I must have seen time and again on the walls in the museums back in Italy—the model female forms of way back when breasts and stomach infused each painter's strokes with passion.

That first night I made my way to my drawer where a bottle of whiskey swayed and sat in front of my new friend, Meagan. I began to feel that freedom even more as she asked me, "So what's your story?"

I could have made up anything in that moment I looked back at her, swallowing back the notion that perhaps I could begin to weave a tale—one that involved health and happiness. I could introduce myself as a new version of me. I could invent a tale of me and him that I hadn't already done to Dan, to Jessie, to my doctors, to anyone back home who knew me and my family. And in that tale, I'd only include the moments that I loved.

"Oh, me? Well, nothing really. Flavia works at Boeing and just moved home. She's twenty-two. Finance major—type A. Then there's

Nicole. She's twelve. Really sweet and gifted. She's always sticking up for me. My parents are Italian and yeah, I'd say the stereotypes are all correct—" I could have said with a laugh. And Meagan would have laughed back, before eating some popcorn I prepared.

And it would have been true. Even if my mother and father were out spending an August morning in the square, drinking a cappuccino in the Piazza del Popolo beside a wrought-iron table—or a round, white plastic table with matching white chairs. Hearing the bell chimes from the church just feet away from where they sat, and Don Peppe walking up on their right from Vico Diritto, his back hunched over and his face red and glistening.

"Buongiorno," my mom would have called out, and my father would have nodded as they'd make eye contact with Don Peppe. And in my made-up memory, Don Peppe says a prayer beneath his breath and my father speaks.

It would have been true—the details I'd invoke, reflecting my desires in that moment when I could have invented a new life. Instead, I skirted the issue of my family and listened to Meagan recount the problems she had with her parents, her fights with her mother, her own gifted younger brother. And so it was that we became close because of our similar depressions. My past with cutting she could identify with; she used to pull out her hair. And when the subject of my father was brought up, she looked at me and grew invisible. I never did respond well to the empathy, remorse or pity I got because of his dementia. Meagan disappears from my dorm room that evening as I try to envision our conversation and my mind floats again towards that home in the Guardiola, down through the stone pathways and the cement-laden walls, the old painting of the virgin beside our neighbor's front doorway laden with beads. I squint my memory towards the window to our kitchen, the small square window where a white curtain sways and around the sounds of my mother mopping the remnants of her husband's urine on the bathroom floor.

But I can't see where he is, I only see him smiling and laughing— that laughter through his throat, that Donald Duck sound he makes with his glasses pushed up on his forehead. I only see his shirt sticking to his back as he stares off into the mountains surrounding the house he no longer understands and back to my mother as she realizes he no longer understands.

WHEN MEAGAN LEFT my room that night, I made my way to bed, up onto my top bunk. My sheets were black and my comforter a dark navy blue. I listened to the sounds of the oscillating fan swirling the hot and humid air over and under the surfaces of my room. I am alone on the bed, and faraway she's lying awake dreading the return flight home—the voyage back and the journey still consuming us.

Chapter 18

My father walked amid a pool of white geese the last time he, my mother and I left the movies on a weekend evening sometime before they set out for their last trip to Pacentro. It was a little chilly I recall, that evening we left the movie, avoiding the crowds and leaving through the back door. It may very well have been the last time he ever did go to a film in a theatre—something he loved to do, something he and my mother loved to do together. Usually, it would be a double feature of some kind, with the thrill of saving a few bucks and taking full advantage of the movie and the price. They were adamant about seeing double features each time they'd see a movie, and the one time they did try a triple feature, my mother explained to me afterwards, "That was just too much—I don't think we'll do that again . . ."

So that night we left, after just *one* movie, leaving through the back door away from the crowd. My mother, I believe it was, pushed the heavy door and held it open as I walked quickly through, and then my father. And there they were—a pillow of white, squawking in all shades of harmony, some walking, some sitting, some crossing the pathway in front of us. We laughed, my mother and I, and I turned to look at him, the silent one, and heard that laugh of his through his nose and in his throat and saw through the moonlight that sparkle in his eyes.

He stood among the geese, my dad in his jeans barely fastened across his growing belly, his untucked polo tee-shirt and a light jacket. His feet scuttled across the way in his sneakers, the laces tied tight thanks to one of us back home who dressed and prepared him for this evening out. The geese gathered around him like he was their god, their leader. And he just laughed and smiled, looking up at us, and down once more, at the wild white geese.

ON THE PLANE ride coming back from Pacentro that summer in 2002, my father would have dropped his white pillow onto the seat or on the floor as my mother grabbed his arm to hold him steady as the flight attendant came near.

"I need to take him to the bathroom," she told the flight attendant that afternoon they flew across the Atlantic. Dropping her voice, my mother said to her, "He has Alzheimer's disease. I have to help him."

I wonder what the flight attendant thought as she led the way to the bathroom, watching as my mother kept the door open, pulling down his pants, holding him steady and pushing him down onto the seat. "I'll give you some privacy and keep the other passengers away until you're through," she said to my mother, who still remembers the strain and the trouble it was trying to keep him in line and calm.

And when she was through and had gotten him settled back into his seat, the white pillow edged between his skin and cushion, the flight attendant took my mother in her arms and embraced her. "I'm so sorry," she told my mother, as my father sat looking somewhere past them, somewhere we couldn't see—a place somehow set within a time or a place that he only knew and hopefully understood. He was experiencing life totally separate from us by then, and no amount of aid or compassion could settle him—because he was angry and confused, agitated and not himself.

When they landed, he sat in a wheelchair just as his mother had when she visited us that year they got arrested. It was the day Flavia and I drove around looking for a certain movie theatre we would go to when he was well. We thought we had seen it from the highway, its green rooftop just to the left of us—it was just a ways down. But when we finally got to it, we realized it was just a random green-roofed building somewhere in the city. We had to stop at a gas station and Flavia tried to keep calm, but she was nervous. She hadn't been driving long and never had she driven alone in the city. And I was no help. I had been the one pressuring her to keep following that building—confident that it was the movie theatre.

By the time we made it back home, a few hours had passed. "I can't believe Nicole didn't come with us," Flavia said to me, worried and regretful. "I would have taken her with us—I just can't understand her sometimes."

"Fla—I think she's just used to the fighting—" I piped in.

"Well that's worse than anything else, Stef. If that's the case—that's not normal at all."

And when we pulled up to the house that day, they were gone, and the voicemail played with Linda's normally light and feathery voice resounding in a fearful tone—"Hey, Flavia? When you get home, come to my house. Your sister and your grandma are here. . . . "

Finding myself crying on her flowery sofa chair in the living room, I didn't seem to notice that Flavia wasn't beside me like she was before when the music was blaring from the radio and our laughter was the only other sound besides the wind beating against the windows.

MY MOM WALKED beside my father, who was pushed by an airport worker. My father was angry that moment—probably from the strain of the flight and the fact that he couldn't move and walk around and around like he had grown used to.

I imagine he had the same look of disdain on his face that his mother had when he and I went to pick her up that day at the airport. We had arrived late because my father always seemed to run late, and we came upon her darkened scowl as she sat uncomfortably in a wheelchair. She was being pushed by a man in an airport uniform—an indiscriminate aide come to perform his duty of pushing handicapped patients, elderly patients, in wheelchairs down the busy halls of the airport.

She was by then completely surrendered to the effects of her dementia—though only my mother knew it for certain. It was only my mother again who had called his brother, Zio Mario, and received the embittered tone of disbelief and anger at her accusations that his brother too had come across the same fate as his mother.

But all of this is just a loosened strand in the carpet caught on another creak and squeak of the wheels straining, the leather seat sinking. All of it beneath the weight of my father's dementia that day my mother stood beside him as he was pushed alongside her down the halls of the airport.

"And then we finally got to the entrance to have our passports checked," she told me over the phone after I asked her about the trip back. "And he slapped me across the face." I already know the pity in her eyes and the understanding she showed him afterwards. I can hear through her pauses, the description of the airport aide that came to her and looked at him accusingly. I can see the way she turned to the guard who didn't know her or my father, and I can see the way her mouth moves over the words, "It's OK—he's sick."

And I see the way the guard nods, understanding her when she says he has Alzheimer's disease, seeing an image of a grandfather, a grandmother, and then looking once over at the man in a fifty-year-old frame and the unhinged mind inside of it.

WHEN MY PARENTS finally arrived home from Italy, I had to wait until the weekend to go and see them. I had been spending most of my time with Meagan, sharing secrets and affection. She was my steady source of comfort. I had been keeping in touch with Dan as well. He was in Florida—after having mistakenly applied to Tallahassee instead of Tampa. Needless to say, Dan had pulled a "Dan" and his procrastination had led him to a town he would not have otherwise chosen. Jessie had gone to Missouri Baptist and it was just as fitting. I was looking forward to seeing her again that weekend I would go home and visit my parents.

As my roommate pulled into my driveway that Friday early evening to drop me off, I said goodbye without a hint of desperation. I jumped out of the passenger seat, grabbed my bag and ran towards the garage.

"Ma?!" I yelled out into the empty kitchen, darkened by the shadows streaming in from the branches of the trees hanging over the deck. "Ma? Nicole?" I asked again, sure I'd hear Nicole running up the stairs of the basement, excited to see me.

"Fla?" Maybe Flavia would be the one excited to see me. I hadn't been home in a few weeks, and we had talked on the phone often since I'd been away at my school, my studying, and anything else. She and I had become closer since she had moved me to college. I had started seeing her differently ever since she selflessly gave herself to me and my every need that afternoon.

"Stefa? I'm outside. Come here!" I heard my mom's voice coming from outside on the deck.

"Hi, Ma. I missed you," I said, as I kissed her on the cheek and hugged her.

"Did you see your father?" she asked as I stood in front of her, squinting a bit from the light of the setting sun.

"No, where is he?"

"He's inside the family room. Go see him," she said without looking at me.

I turned away quickly and made my way to the family room, to his green recliner that sat unextended. I could see his arm bent, his palm holding his chin as he sat facing the television. I don't imagine the TV was even on. No, I see it off, the shades I see were mainly closed as my father sat alone.

And I went quickly to him. "Dad? Daddy?" I stood in front of him and immediately tears welled into my eyes as I saw my father remarkably changed after only about a month of not seeing him. He had gained weight and when I went to embrace him, he hardly even responded.

"Daddy—I missed you," I said to him as I tried to force his arms around me. In the end, I think I only managed to kiss his cheek and run my hand lightly over his own bent arm. I went quickly to my mother, leaving my emotionless father alone again to sit and ponder in that suffocating family room.

"He's changed, mom! He's so different," I cried. "I don't understand how he could change so much! He didn't even smile! He hardly looked at me!" I kept saying, over and over again as my mother sat quietly, every so often telling me, "I know, Stefa—I know it's hard."

"How could he have changed *so* much in that short a time!? I don't understand." I felt as though I had unwillingly let go of another layer of my father.

"It's OK, Stefania. What are you gonna do?" My mother lay back into the patio chair. Leaning her head back against the white cushion, she raised her closed eyes up towards the sky. "I gotta wash this deck—it's so filthy."

AT HOME, HELP came to my mother—to all of us—more readily. More willingly, it seemed, and more gently. What was once the hardest decision my mother had yet to face—whether or not to move back to her town, to their town, and hopefully find themselves nestled in with the familiar scents and sounds, the breath of the pallid stones and her hope for peace—was now no more. She was confident she had made the right choice.

It was Jessie's mother who happened to come right at the moment when my father grew to be completely incontinent. He had peed more frequently on the floor in Pacentro—and when he arrived home from the trip that fall, he had developed a tendency to grow severely agitated, more so than usual, walking around and around the kitchen and the family room, right past the door to the bathroom.

My mom had taught me to ask my dad during these times if he had to go to the bathroom. I was alone with him downstairs one afternoon when he was doing just that—growing tenser. I thought he was surely about to explode.

"Daddy? Dad? Do you have to use the bathroom? Do you?" I asked him as I followed him up and down the hallway to the kitchen and back to his chair in the family room. Finally, after no response, I led him to the bathroom and pushed down his pants. I kept my eyes on his face, too scared to look down.

And I knew I could just sit him down on the seat because I had watched my mom do it other times before. But what I didn't know was that I had to make sure his penis aimed downwards into the toilet. I had simply just sat him down and told him, "OK, daddy. OK you can go."

When he peed all over the small carpet in front of the toilet and his urine made its way to the edge of the door, I yelled upstairs for my mom to come and help me, while he just sat still for a second longer before standing again, his pants at his ankles.

"Goddamnit, Stefania!" She screamed, "You are so stupid! God-damnit!" She cried, completely crazed and out of control; she tried to slap me, and I ran away crying. She couldn't believe what I had done—or hadn't done, really.

And if that was the worst part for me, the day Flavia had to wash his own stool from his body in the shower may have been the worst for her. He had had an accident of a different kind, and Flavia was alone with him—and alone, still, with a memory she refuses to give up, unlock, and relive again.

So when Jessie's mother came into our lives with the diapers, my mother eagerly assented to the help—and I knew as I shut the trunk of the Volvo that it was time to accept all forms of help that came our way as well.

I would email Jessie often from school—poetry and dreams I'd have, all of them about him. In one dream I sent her, I am asleep in my bed, awakened by the silhouette of my father standing in the doorway. He creeps inside and lies beside me. He cries, and I hold him. We become quiet; I hear his softened breathing as he falls into sleep. Instead, I feel two, three jumps, and suddenly he remains lifeless and empty. And I feel guilt—that he should die in my own arms and not in those of my mother.

I always received some kind of response from Jessie that had to do with faith. She was so spiritual and I would hunger for the words she'd offer me. One day, she sent me a passage from the Bible. Instantly, I felt a bit unnerved and turned off. Though I was beginning to let go of my deep despair—my tendency towards hating everything— receiving a Bible verse was still something I couldn't receive without gagging—even if just slightly.

This is what I received from Jessie one night as I sat on my dorm room floor that fall: "So we fix our eyes not on what is seen, but on what is unseen. For what is seen is temporary, but what is unseen is eternal" (2 Corinthians 4:18).

My roommate also liked to read the Bible—mainly at night before bed. She, a sorority girl, tall and beautiful with Winnie Cooper hair. And at night, almost every night, she'd put on her retainer, her glasses and cozy up with her Bible. After Jessie sent me the verse, I had my roommate read aloud to me from her Bible. We decided to write it in large block letters on white paper and tape it to our wall that faced our bunk beds. From the top bunk, I felt it sort of kept me safe—at least from falling out of bed at night.

JESSIE TOLD ME in an email, or perhaps it was over the phone, that her mother could help my mom with medical supplies if ever the need should arise. I never really understood what part her mother played in the medical-supply field—all I know is that her office had a desk beside a large fish tank. Jessie's mom had Jessie's broad smile, and eyes that squinted when she laughed.

I parked my Volvo station wagon in the parking lot of her mother's office the day after my mother called her, telling her she really could use her help after all. I remember walking towards the doors with Jessie by my side. The sky was gray and it looked like it might rain as

I opened the door and saw the fish tank before I saw her.

She had saved several boxes of adult diapers and helped me put them in my car. I think she got them wholesale and sold them. In any case, these diapers would be free for my mother. Somewhere inside of him, I'm sure my dad must have been happy about that.

"Tell your mother to call me if she needs anything else. I swear—I can get pretty much anything if she lets me know before hand. I . . . I am really sorry, Stefania," she said as she went towards me and hugged me harder than I thought she could.

"Thank you so much—" I said, and stopped. I spitefully slammed the trunk shut on several cases of diapers he would now have to wear. I was almost starting to get used to that feeling.

AFTER WE GOT him the diapers, he peed on the bathroom floor much less, though my mother didn't always keep him in diapers. So the accidents still came. I was coming home as many weekends as I could that first semester, hoping I wouldn't see such a big change as I had that summer. On one afternoon, I was downstairs in the family room with him. He was sitting at the edge of his recliner, seconds away from sliding off and walking towards the dining room, the living room, the kitchen. He would stumble off that chair momentarily, I knew it. I tried hard to watch the television with him "Dad—look! Dad? You like this show—" trying to distract him and make those angered eyes calm down just a bit. But his face always seemed tense and his look would be one of worry every day he'd make his repetitive track from his chair, to the living room, to the front door, to the dining room, to the kitchen, to the bathroom and again into the family room. I'd let him go alone until I'd hear a crash or hear a silence that would last too long. I'd imagine him rummaging in the drawers, or getting out chocolate again or eating scraps off the floor.

But that one afternoon, he kept wincing, kept crying out, kept limping. My mother and sisters and I yelled at him—"Shut up! Just sit down! Just stop it!" And just like every other day, he wouldn't listen and would just keep going. It was like he was being led by a string someone had tied to the edge of his skin—every jerk and pull so painful and so powerful that he was helpless to stop it. He had to move, had to jerk and jump and wince and cry because he couldn't get free. He was a human lure under that disease, but that afternoon, he was something else as well. Something else had a grip over him and we were all so used to his cries, we remained indifferent, if not annoyed.

We found out a few days later, after a doctor's appointment, that he had had a kidney stone. Nicole, I remember, was the most vocal, "I can't believe we didn't believe him! Poor daddy!" she cried, and inside my mind I kept envisioning myself as eight and afraid of all the spiders in our basement.

We lived in Omaha, Nebraska, when I was in second grade, for the 1991-1992 school year. My dad was receiving his over-the-hill birthday cards—the perks of being in his early forties, I guess. And within the memories I have between the sleepovers with friends, the second-grade glue eaters and my First Communion, is a vision of the spiders in the basement bathroom.

I had just taken a shower, and I was excited to be using the new bathroom in the basement. The paint still smelled fresh and the tile in the shower was white and shiny like pearls surrounding me on all sides. As I stepped out of the shower and reached for my towel, I saw the spiders crawling on the wall—the ceiling, too. I must have thought I saw twenty in an instant, but really there was only one, maybe two. And they were nothing more than daddy long legs, but that didn't stop me from screaming and running out nearly naked onto the carpeted area before the stairs.

I heard him moaning before I saw him.

He was on the sofa, lying on his back, expressing such pain in such awful sounds I had never heard from him before. It was almost as painful as the moment I first saw him cry, the day he got the phone call that his father had died.

He had nothing but his own limited devices scavenging about the house looking for appeasement. I saw the spiders first and then heard his moans that day I realized we had left him in pain.

AFTER THE DIAPERS came the hospital bed that my mother put in the dining room. "I thought it would let him sleep better—not having to go up those stairs. I thought he would lie down more."

The men who brought the bed parked it in the dining room so that it lay against the wall. My mom must have had them help her move the heavy carved and ornamented chest that stood in its place. She must have quickly gathered the candles that sat atop it; the white, hand-stitched lace tablecloth that I used to lift to dust beneath as a young teenager must have surely had a stain when she finally removed the silver tray from atop it. I can see her carelessly tossing them on the dining room table. Maybe Nick Rallo came to help her; Linda may have brought little Nicholas. And in the room at the other side of the house, in the family room near his chair, I can almost see his eyes following Nicholas' meandering steps until they lock eyes and share a secret between friends.

The final adjustment of the bed, the linens she took from the closet upstairs—twin size to fit the mattress—and the way her hand must have swept across the surface of the sheets after she tucked the corners in—I can see it all so clearly as though it all had happened just like that.

But then I remember that all I really did see was the bed and the door to the dining room left ajar. I remember having a friend or two over and hoping they'd see the bed and know that something awful was coming, had come and was now gone.

HE NEVER LAY in that bed. And if he did, he'd get right back up again and try to move around again, frantic and crazed. If he were somewhere else, and someone else too—maybe a man searching for his child in a tower that was burning down, maybe a mother fighting for her baby's safe return to her arms again, maybe even just a man again with something pressing and important to get done—then it would have all made sense. Those other scenarios could have been warranted, expected—normal. But as I lay in my bed, awake, staring at my ceiling that still sparkled with the specks of glow-in-the-dark lights shining from the stars I had stuck on the ceiling, I could hear her shrieks.

She had reached the breaking point. Ties were left on the railings. In the mornings, I would sometimes see them coupled with her drawn face that would turn into screams at any point for any problem or any air of scent or sound.

He was sent to a hospital to adjust his medicine on the 27th of December 2002. It may have been the second or third time my mother took him to the geriatrics floor of the hospital downtown. It was the same building Dan and I passed on our drives to The Grind. Barnes Jewish. It was the same hospital that stood tall, lit and stationary as the years swept by within my car and Dan's. Laughing and singing—one night it would be to a band we loved, another, a musical made entirely of naked men singing (it was Dan's latest find), and another in silence. Such were the drives Dan and I took that first semester in college whenever I would visit. And such was that evening my mother took my father to the hospital to stay and be realigned in a way—to be readjusted.

I visited once when he was there. And it frightened me more than I thought it would. A hospital. A wing dedicated to the elderly infirm. And there, in the small waiting room, or living room, or maybe it was a sitting room, he sat behind the glass windows. He was among several old women and men, and for the first time I felt an inkling of the absurdity of it all. But I only got an inch of it because before I knew it, I was being whisked away with my mother and sisters and he was being put to bed by a doctor who said, "His dementia is certainly getting worse."

I wanted to tell this doctor and all the nurses there to go to hell with your observations of this crazed man in your old, withered wing.

Give him the pills to make him calm again, to make him sleep again, and maybe my mother will finally calm down again.

But we left him there that night and we walked towards the elevators. We still had Christmas bells to avoid and cheer and Santa's taunting laugh on the radio that was quickly switched to music. Italian music, of course. But if Nicole were in the car, with her ever-growing authority in her booming voice, the radio would have been switched to music of her liking, while the rest of us either fought her on it or gave up the fight of feeling.

I find myself always lying awake in bed and staring at the ceiling during these toughest moments and these clearest moments of when he changed the most. And always, I am in my mind away from others even if I hear them calling my name. Even if I hear them fighting or my father moaning or my mother wailing, I find I always tried my hardest to keep myself in my room alone in the dark. And those small fragments of light from my ceiling that slowly faded away were the only bits of intrusion that I seemed to accept without question.

I try and wonder now when it was that I first pondered the questions that really matter, the ones that make a story meaningful. The questions that serve the purpose of giving life a purpose. I recall only focusing on the reasons for how and why that echoed behind each length of his faltering steps. The ideas of how and why don't matter once it's happened—it's happened. I must have had to ask myself over and again these two questions before I was able to move past it. That's probably where my true weakness lay. The how and the why prompted me again and again to stare outside my window, to shake the glass over the melting ice cubes, to slash one more time in a spot better hidden. To cry tears for a boy I loved and who suddenly stopped loving me back. To withstand the sounds I heard from outside my doorway, of his forgetting and her last few senses giving way before the bridge would break and he would be left on one side while we waved goodbye on the other.

When was it that I lay motionless and speechless, trying to figure out what this journey really was? How long did it take for me to start wondering how much time I really had left with him? How much time *he* had left with us? I try now to see if in the seconds where time seems to whisper these memories to me in waves, if I ever really questioned what the meaning was of it all? And why did my father have to lose himself in order for *us* to find it?

We stood beside a mountain, and I wonder when it was that I realized I had to climb it in order to get beyond it. Here was strength, and if I could grab a hold of even just a piece of it—withstand the jagged edges and my bleeding palms—I could move forward. We could move forward and we could do so together.

But if I know my nineteen-year-old self at all, I know she wasn't yet asking those questions. I see through her eyes, the glow-in-the-dark stars and fragments slowly fading into the blackness of her room, and I know for sure that any other light that was dimming elsewhere, she simply wouldn't and couldn't seem to accept.

Because I still imagined sometimes, sitting on the sofa, evenings and late afternoons, I'd still imagine there was a time not too long ago, and possibly another time returning, of me and him just sitting. Watching TV. Just sitting like we used to in one of my earliest memories—me when I was four or three, eating pork rinds on the couch beside him. Just a snippet of recollection of the two of us on that gray couch that we later kept in the basement where Nicole would watch television every day after school. It was on that couch that we watched *Three's Company*, laughing at things I didn't quite understand but faking it to make him think I did.

And it was what he did the best. The faking part—the faking at understanding. Though I know, somewhere inside him, he still understood.

There is a moment before the hospital bed, before the diapers. Though it was after my worst parts, my screams at him to leave me alone, my misplaced hate. Yes, it must have been right before his last trip to Pacentro that I remember sitting on our green leather couch in the family room, not eating but sitting still. My arms and legs resting against his; me snuggling my head into his arm, acting as a small child would, the little girl who used to bounce on his knee promising him that she'd never marry.

It was in a lull between his pacing and his resting that I caught him on the sofa and sat down right beside him. He was staring at the television screen on some channel left on from before. He was fake-watching the TV probably, according to the doctor. But I thought he was watching it just fine—to me, he even seemed bored by the channel. So, after doing some flipping, I found the perfect show for the perfect moment. It was his favorite show that I found— *Sanford and Son.* Satisfied and even proud for finding it, I put his arm around my shoulder and leaned against him lightly. I laughed out loud on purpose at the funny parts and looked at him. I watched his burrowed eyes lighten and his taught mouth give way to a chuckle.

But the moment washes up on the shore before me that night we left him at the hospital. We drove home thinking it was a temporary separation, just to set him on track again. We all must have known—even I must have known we were beginning something new. My mother, Flavia, Nicole and myself—we had all spent almost four years standing with him, holding him up and fighting what was now fast approaching.

And as the wind whipped by our car that night as we drove home, we couldn't yet see our white flag flailing in the shadows above us.

PART IV

Fall 2002 - Summer 2004

Chapter 19

I wonder if, beside my foot, his ashes shook as we made our way across the roads that lead up the mountain. I wonder if I held my breath as my uncle sped across the lanes of traffic the moment I spotted the sign that read "Pacentro" and the kilometers still left for us to traverse.

I was running out of time. From then, I could precisely calculate the minutes I had left, imagining the rest of the roads and the turns we'd still have to take. From then on, I knew exactly what the pathway was ahead of us and it shook me even harder than before—because I knew now what was coming. I was going to be saying a final goodbye.

But now as I write those words I seem to see only glimpses and hear only certain sounds: the whirring of the car, my mother's murmurs into the wind and perhaps even the smell of my uncle's cigarette.

Memory, *my* memory, works within visions and sounds and scents, light and dark shades of people and places coalescing and swelling as in the ocean, within the changing waters of our past. I stand beside my sisters and my mother before the sea, looking out at him diving into the shallow waves as we stand atop the sand.

Now when I look into the car that afternoon, the sunlight first catches my attention, then the wind and then my hair streaming and dancing, flailing, more likely, into the air. I don't recall if we traveled on that road that intersects one leading to Sulmona and another that leads into my mother's sister, Zia Cristina's town—a town called Pettorano. Back behind her home, one grand mountain superimposes itself on the others that lie behind it. The views are still majestic, yet the mountains seem to become one. Looking out from my aunt's backyard, the town's borders seem to face one side of a mountain that eclipses the range of those beyond. There seem to be fewer views of the rolling mountain range that softly serenade Pacentro, pulsating a beauty I attempt to unfold.

On the other side of the intersection, the road takes you to the ocean, to the towns that approach the cliffs that surround the Adriatic Sea. Somewhere along that road, up to where it meets the highway, Flavia and Nicole were driving. I like to think they were singing loudly in their car—laughing over the parts they fumbled and stumbled over together.

There is another way to reach Pacentro—one from the highway, the autostrada we undoubtedly took from Rome. But I can't recall too many specifics of that road—I only see it now at dusk from when I was six years old and my father first told me his memory of falling.

I will choose to see us in the car now, riding across that intersection, past the road to Pettorano, past the road to Flavia and Nicole. As the car hurried across the lanes of traffic before entering the path that would lead us up the mountain, I would have felt the shadows of the trees, seen the lines of the railings of the balconies—I may have even seen their shadows on my arms, on my hands, as we began our ascent.

Yes, I would have been entwined in shadows and feeling panic rising inside of me as I would have looked down again at my foot. I would have looked for only a second before I'd turn my eyes upwards, up past the trees and the houses, up over the rooftop terraces and over the sounds of the engine that indelibly morphed into a high-pitched "beep."

I HAD HEARD the alarm sound and a mumbled "hello" come from my side. There, two nurses' aides were standing behind a desk, monitoring the common area that lay before them. Following their gaze, I spotted another nurse sitting in a large circle in the common room, surrounded by a white mass of slouching women, drooling moans and closing eyes. I saw but two men within the group, and a large, colored rubber ball roll slowly within their circle.

This was my first glimpse into the nursing home; the place we had feared for so long was now in front of me.

Minutes before, my mother had arrived in front of Bethesda's large, sliding glass doors. She sat in the backseat with my father as her friend drove her in. I don't know if it was Linda—though it may have been someone else. It really doesn't matter who drove them—only that they all were there. When my father was at the hospital, the doctors said it was time that he should go to a nursing home. My mother says they were worried about her mental state—as well as Nicole's. Nicole was just twelve at the time and with adolescence now engulfing her, the doctors wanted her to keep neurosis at bay. To keep the sadness that had enveloped me away.

I don't imagine my mother could have decided this on her own. I would have fought it for sure. When Flavia had taken me out for a drive one afternoon, she had said, "Stef, you know dad is probably gonna go to a nursing home soon, right?"

"What!" I screamed, nearly swerving. I continued, "What the hell for? You're home! He's not that bad yet!"

"Stef, are you kidding me? Are you serious? Mom is going crazy— we all are. I am! He needs more help—"

And I kept driving, more angry and more anxious—eventually Flavia had to drop it after realizing I couldn't even handle the thought of it.

But that afternoon—it came and it was as real as the sound of the passenger door slamming shut as my mother held my father arm in arm and waited for the nurse to greet them with a wheelchair.

My mother says she only agreed to send him right from the hospital on one condition—"I told them *I* wanted to take him. I told them no ambulance—just me."

And so, on January 8, 2003, she got her wish as she pushed us aside and grabbed the handle bars behind him, as he sat, hopefully, not knowing where it was he was being led.

I had hoped he wouldn't know—especially the second I saw the common area, the taut and emotionless faces—and that ridiculous beach ball.

FOR A MOMENT I waited, standing stiffly, as far away from that circle in the common area as I could be. My mother began speaking to the nurses, signing papers, preparing. I looked down at my father, who was sitting in a wheelchair at her side, and his eyes were closed.

He was scared, I remember thinking. Or rather, I was. I was standing apart from the rest of those people in the room—standing separately from the patients with my mom, sisters and my dad. We kept our distance in those first few moments, after the shock of where we were hit us. The shock reverberated from the walls of the nursing home, the white of the patients and the deafening fact that we could no longer help him on our own. But really, for the past seven years since he'd been ill, his mind decaying slowly within him, all I could do, really, was watch. I felt utterly helpless. I don't think I ever really believed that he would come to this. Yet, there he was beside my mother, who stood signing him away from us to the nurses.

Not long after, she turned towards my father's wheelchair and grabbed a hold of the black handles. She looked straight ahead of herself as she pushed him down the white tiled floor between the nurses' station and the common area. I walked slowly behind her, but suddenly, I was stuck within myself; I couldn't breathe. I didn't have the energy to move and I didn't see, or rather didn't *want* to see any damn reason for us to be there.

I felt dizzy looking around me—felt my head, heavy, dripping, drowning in my memory, realizing the air was just as suffocating. Why were we here? Am I next? Why am I thinking of me? I often felt the moments of fear and panic tear through me. I would bury it further down inside of me, because I knew at least for now, that I was not the victim. My dad was. I entered the nursing home that day and I already feared the fate of so many grandfathers and so many grandmothers. I feared my life would be cut short, just like my dad's was.

And as these thoughts raced through my mind, I tasted the tears that fell in torrents down my cheeks. I had to leave, so I quickly turned around. I left the sounds of the heavy, squeaking wheels of my father's wheelchair—sounds that followed me, sickened me with their slow persistence, a slow, jagged saw caressing the strings of a violin.

Why could I not handle this moment of his deep descent? I knew somewhere inside him he knew where he was. Did he always know he was coming here? Did he know he'd come to this? I surely didn't. Yet my mom always tried to warn me. That day as a twisted and tainted teenager, I'll never forget what I felt reading that stapled bundle of paper my mother threw at me—that day I learned he would one day lose his smile.

Having left the procession of walking my father down to his new bedroom, I turned quickly towards those double doors beside the nurses' station. I heard my mom and sisters call for me but I ignored them. "I'll be the one who's afraid," I thought to myself.

I felt eyes prickling my skin and suddenly felt a light hand like an insect laid upon my arm. I jumped and turned to face a startled woman with dark brown hair pulled back into a bun.

"Get me outta here!" she yelled.

I shook my head at her and panicked. Looking up at the nurses who sat emotionless behind the desk, I wondered if they even noticed we were there.

When I tried to open the double doors to leave the unit, I found them locked. I gasped as I sensed that woman hovering behind me. There was a number pad needing a security code in order to unlock the doors. Of course, in that instant, I didn't know the code and was fumbling, trying desperately to flee from that ward.

As my fingers shook and I began feeling anxious, I imagined if this sense of fear was what my father must have felt those days the numbers started leaving him. The nurses must have seen me struggling, so they yelled out the code for me. And as I finally got the numbers right, I felt the blood rush down my face and chest. I quickly stepped out and heard the nurses call out to me to shut the door quickly. As I turned to make sure the door would latch, I caught a glimpse of that woman who had scared me with her touch, with her crazed expression—"Please, I need to leave," she said.

I heard the doors latch and stood there. I shut my eyes tightly. I kept seeing the circle of those patients in their nightgowns. I kept seeing the smile of the nurse within the circle, passing that giant ball around, nodding at them and prodding them. I rubbed my forehead as I raised my eyes, and turned myself around. I stood facing the two beige doors, the little black sign that read "Alzheimer Unit."

It was treacherous—that struggle to leave the unit. I had to dodge the indifferent nurses, bypass that crazy woman. When my dad ran away from home that afternoon, did he face any such obstacles? Did he panic?

I wanted to run now, too. I wanted to run back in time to when this day was nothing but a stage I read about in that packet of paper.

Exhaling, I took a few steps away from the doors. There was weakness I felt but there was also that fear. What if I couldn't handle this new level of my father's affliction? I was so angry, angry at being there, angry at those people sitting sickly in a circle. I was angry my mother had to push my father as he sat nearly comatose in his young skin. I just wanted to go back in time to those days when I was a child, just a few years back in time.

I know it wasn't as if we had a perfect family, a perfect past with perfect times I can happily recall on a whim. But it's in the small cracks and crevices where the air gets through, enlivening an otherwise hollow space, that my family excelled the best. In those little gushes of air, like that evening my dad got spaghetti sauce on the back of his neck, after my mother made him wear a napkin tucked into his collar— "Giovan—that's Ralph Lauren. Put that napkin on!" After he was finished eating and my mother came around him to help him fix his collar, she had seen the sauce and started laughing. We all had. "You see? I'm always right," my mom had said, as she quickly took his soiled shirt to the laundry room.

I wanted those family moments. Just like the times of my father's worst moments, the best memories were just as fluid. Yet again, I wanted something I couldn't have. My hand still shook as I pushed the doors open and went back inside.

MY FATHER'S ROOM had two twin beds and a curtain hanging in between. This curtain acted as a makeshift wall between two patients living side by side. Thankfully, my dad had no roommates—at least for now. He was one of three men in the Alzheimer unit, and the men all got their own separate rooms. My dad was lying on the bed closest to the windows. My mom was busying herself by unpacking his clothes into drawers, refolding his tee shirts and sweatpants, and commanding my sisters and me every so often to hang another pair of pants in the closet. I watched my dad as he lay there atop the mauve and pink comforter of his bed, not moving, not making a sound.

After a while, my mother finished unpacking his life into drawers and had sat down beside my dad when a pair of narrowed, nearly black, dark blue eyes in tortoise-framed glasses met us from the doorway. She entered my dad's room strongly and her presence dominated every space and every bit of air in the room. She walked slowly towards where I was sitting and I thought I surely must have been mistaken—her anger must have been my imagination.

She creaked into the room, limping a bit as she asked me, "Patty, when can you come tomorrow?"

I looked blankly at her—and grabbed my father's hand tighter.

"No, no. No party tomorrow. We have to discuss your decision. You can bring the girls if you like," she continued. She was closer to me at this point, and I could see her eyes looking straight into mine like needles I felt penetrating my pupils.

"And do not forget to wash these shoes," she said as she placed a pair of white loafers by my side. The heels were worn and the soles were dirtied from years of use—perhaps years within these walls, up and down the tiled hallways.

I looked harder into her eyes without squinting. Timidly nodding my head in agreement, I told her, "OK, yes."

She was satisfied by my answer and nodded. Her eyes seemed distant as they tore away from my own and grazed the top of my head. After our talk, I noticed how their color had changed to a lighter shade of blue behind her large glasses.

"OK Patty. Bye-bye. Let me give you a kiss at least," she said as she stooped down towards where I was sitting.

I held my cheek up towards her and closed my eyes. When she was gone, I looked around the room. My mom and sisters were laughing and looking at each other, commenting on that woman who had just stormed in. I looked down at her shoes sitting there on the bed, quiet and small.

Not long after, she reappeared in the doorway. Her faded eyes were ocean swells, and angry. Her limp was stronger as she approached me—

"Well, who are you? *Child of damnation*! I need to know where Patty is!"

She left just as suddenly as her mood had changed. I caught my breath in a gasp, feeling frightened and alone. I didn't know why I was the only one reacting in such a way. Why couldn't I laugh it off as my sisters and mother had? My father was looking at all of us, yet I was sure he hadn't seen the woman who had just left. I wanted him to protect me from these patients and these prisoners.

A nurse came inside the bedroom, her smile a bit too broad and her red, wavy hair pulled back tightly in a ponytail. "Oh, I'm very sorry for that interruption before. That woman was Adeline Kirby. She likes to pretend that this is her room. She gets confused sometimes. I'm very sorry," she said. "It's actually time for dinner if you all want to take John to the common area."

We thanked the nurse for coming in to tell us about that woman—Adeline Kirby—and we told her we'd be in for dinner shortly.

My mother helped my dad out of bed. He looked around the room and down at his feet. He had on a new pair of slippers that he would have to wear each day. He had to begin to get used to them.

As my mom walked my dad towards the common room, I lagged behind. I walked slowly after my family while taking in everything around me. I eyed a woman who sat with her head slammed against the table, her white fluff of hair sitting on top, her walker at her side. I could hear her moaning.

I smelled the food the servers were handing out to the patients. I could see the shapes upon the plates and the cups of juice before each placemat. I heard nurses calling out different names of patients who sat firmly on recliners lined up in the back of the room. They looked spiteful yet empty, sitting still on those big brown chairs. I spotted a man who was frowning deeply, his face flushed. He was holding hands with a woman next to him in a chair. She, too, frowned as she stared straight before her. They sat weakly beside one another, holding one another's hand as though that were the only thing that made sense to them.

I looked to see where my dad had been seated and was surprised to find him sitting across from Adeline at a small table.

"What's wrong with him? Is he going to eat his food?" Adeline said with disdain, shaking her head as she returned to her own plate of food. "Can I have your Jell-O? —My food tastes like wood-fiber," she continued after a moment—her tone still tinged with total and utter disgust.

As my mother began to cut my father's food for him, I looked up to see an elderly woman with frizzy, light brown hair. She was sitting in a large cushy chair against a wall that faced my father. Her glasses were thick, her eyes a light gray blue, and her mouth was the biggest in the unit. "Operator! Operator!" she yelled, then a second later, began laughing to herself as she ate her food.

"Oh that's just Cleda—Cleda Dubin. She used to be an Operator. I think sometimes she sees herself there," said a heavyset woman with light brown hair in a high ponytail. She had kind eyes and an easy smile—I was instantly drawn to her.

Everyone in the common area finished eating at different times. I watched a few nurses who were chatting amongst themselves, feeding the few who were too still and sickly to feed themselves. Adeline and Cleda were not one of them.

From across the room, I watched a quiet woman sit. She had her napkin on her lap and chewed elegantly, with her mouth closed. She seemed aware of what she was eating—something about her didn't match the others. Maybe it was the way she held her knife and fork so naturally. Her steady strokes while she was cutting her food, or the perfect timing her mouth would open as she'd raise her fork. She looked at her tablemates from to time, as though it were out of habit from dinners she'd share with her family and friends.

I was not the only one who felt uncomfortable sitting in the common room, waiting for nothing to happen. I could tell my sisters were still unsure, my mother—I could see she was trying hard to stay calm and take the lead. At this point, my dad was lucid enough to know he was somewhere else. He looked about the room, looked up at his new kitchen table and instead of sitting there with us, at the head of our familiar table, he sat with a bib around his neck across from Adeline.

We all sat together that evening, huddled in a corner of the common room, taking in our surroundings for the first time, swallowing any bit of defiance we had left. We had to embrace this.

"What's your name?" asked a woman's voice. I looked to my side. I found that small woman I had noticed earlier, who had been eating still and proper from across the room. She was staring at me, the corners of her mouth barely up and smiling. Her teeth were large and protruding from lips that didn't touch. They were a bit like mine, parted and thin. She didn't wear glasses—and her gaze was kind. I believed she was really looking at me this time. Not like that woman, Adeline Kirby, who I heard somewhere in the background, still mumbling about the taste of her food.

"Stefania," I told her.

"Is that your father?" She asked me. She moved her chin towards my father.

"Yes, it is," I answered.

"He's awful young. Why's he here?"

"He's fifty-fifty two. He has Alzheimer's disease." I watched her as I told her, waited for the look of surprise in her eyes, the moment of disbelief and the pity that followed. I welcomed it.

"I'm Wilma," she said. I like to think she winked as she told me, bowing her head as if to say hello.

Wilma and I didn't say much more to each other that first night. But we would, later, at times when she'd sit silently by herself in the common area.

MY MOM FINALLY decided she would take my dad back to his room. I knew we were nearing the end of our time with him. I felt weak and tired—by then, it had been hours since I first left the ward attempting desperately to run away.

I sat again, on that chair in his room, as my mother brushed my dad's teeth and got him ready for bed. Sitting near my sisters in silence, I realized how leaving him there that first night would prove more difficult than taking him there had been.

After my mom put him to bed, my dad looked up at us all as we stood around him. He was lying still and I was thankful. I didn't want the night to end with him agitated. He, too, was tired and I wondered if it was from sadness as well. He looked almost peaceful with his head upon the white, starched pillowcase. My mom had tucked him in tightly, from the night's cold air and the draft of being alone.

And then I saw the tears stream down his cheeks. Where did they come from? I couldn't believe he was crying, that he was, perhaps, aware of us leaving him there. He hadn't spoken all day; he had stayed quiet and listened to us all with attention. Did he believe we were punishing him? Maybe he was scared to be there. Maybe he sensed the fact that he was the youngest by lifetimes in his new home. Maybe he was aware that he was truly sick. Maybe he just knew.

My mother sat beside him on his bed and looked at him. Her eyes were red and glistened as she spoke to him quietly.

"Giovan—this is a hospital. You've got to stay here until you get better. And then I'll take you home."

"Sicuro?" he asked.

"Yes, I'm sure," she responded.

"Sicuro?" he asked again.

"Yeah," she said.

"Prometimi."

"I promise—but you have to behave though—and sit down when they tell you to," she told him.

"I will," he said.

"OK, Giovanni—we'll come back tomorrow," she said, as she got up slowly from the bed.

He lay there, not speaking. He was still. And we left just as quietly.

As we went into the hallway, we looked at one another without saying a word. She had promised him she'd take him home—but we knew it wasn't true. He needed to sleep. Perhaps he needed that piece of hope.

Eventually, I'm sure he'd forgotten that promise my mother made to him as he lay there that first night. That lie made us able to leave him. We believed it too. It made everyone feel better knowing we could change our minds at any time and take him home again. We hadn't realized we were still running away from that disease, even as we shut the door of the Alzheimer unit, got into our car, and drove away.

Chapter 20

The garage door opened slowly as we all sat quietly together in the car. Outside, the air was thick, frigid and mixed with guilt. The January winter had settled and its frigidity had worked its way into each of us, preserving our melancholy as we each closed our doors sharply and walked heavily inside. My mother walked without speaking as she set her coat on the kitchen table, taking off her shoes and leaving them askew on the floor.

"He asked her to promise . . . why? It doesn't make any sense," I thought to myself repeatedly. I hadn't begun to envision a world where he'd be away, but still there. Alive, but not with us. I hadn't imagined a home without him. Though the home I had grown accustomed to was surely not what I had ever envisioned before.

I left Flavia and Nicole downstairs—Flavia had settled somewhere, while Nicole most likely found herself in the basement again. I could see her finding solace in calling a friend, or going on the Internet to chat with friends, or sitting in the company of lamplight and television. I soon found myself in my bedroom, choking on my tightened chest, enveloped with the splash of light reflected from the glow-in-the-dark stars I had put on the ceiling. I stared above, thinking over the day, seeing him in that room, looking up at us with his own tears lightly painting his cheeks in clear, desolate fear and the smell of medicine and the voices from the common area. It was like drowning in thoughts as strong as a current, arms pulling me farther downwards as I panicked for air. I quickly tore the covers away from my body and went into my mother's room.

"Mommy?" I called out to her, childlike and timid. I lay on my father's side of the bed, where I could still feel his indentation. I felt more centered calling for her, as though she acted as both safety and portal to the past— a time when I would lie between them, scooting myself down to their waists so that I could catch them looking at one another. We'd stay that way, until Flavia would lie along our feet and Nicole would join us—then my mother would plan our day and my father would go jogging.

My mother lay beside me with one arm draped over her eyes as she put her other hand out to me, caressing my arm as I cried.

"Stefa . . . I can't do this. No. No, we will take him home in a few days. I just need some time to rest."

And I believed her—she did need time. We all did. We all needed a break from his heavy feet clambering around and around the house, into corners, into closets, around the living room, touching anything he could, swallowing anything he could.

The hospital bed was still in the dining room. Below us it sat, the sheets askew, the pillow still wrinkled, and his necktie hung from the arm bars. He had undeniably regressed to the point of a children's bed, with bars to keep him secure. Even little Nicholas had grown past that stage—it was his turn, then, to sleep in a bed without railings.

"Do you mean it, mom? We'll take him home?" I asked her in between sobs.

"Yes. Just a few days. I can't do this—I can't leave him there," she said, as she grasped my hand and we lay there not speaking for the remainder of the night.

The next morning was more or less the same as usual except my mother was gone, having left before the sun rose that day. Flavia and Nicole were already awake before me, waiting for me to meet them downstairs before leaving for the nursing home.

As WE PULLED into the parking lot, we each spotted our mom's white Volvo parked in the first space, closest to the pathway leading up to the doors. I thought of her arriving before the dawn, in her black coat and boots, her eyes downcast and swollen as she approached the building that morning.

The woman at the front desk looked up at us and smiled—just like yesterday, she showed us that same expression and, again, I felt annoyed. We turned left after her desk, and left once more until we faced the double doors and the sign that read "Alzheimer's Unit." We pressed the red button and waited for the beep and then, just like yesterday, we entered into our father's new *temporary* home.

"Hello, girls!" the heavyset nurse from yesterday, Nurse Patty, said jubilantly. "Your parents are in his room."

As we walked past the nurses' desk beside the door, we looked into the common area, to the women sitting in armchairs lining the windows. We spotted the same man from yesterday, still grasping onto the same woman's hand, his face still flushed, still staring blankly before him. There were tables positioned in the center, and as we passed by them, I saw Wilma sitting at a table near the end with her oxygen tank beside her. She nodded to us and smiled as we passed her. As we approached the hallway to the bedrooms, the white tile beneath fluorescent lights, we could hear Cleda again yelling, "Operator! Operator!" in her squeaky voice, and then shortly afterwards we heard the nurses giggling.

Inside my father's bedroom, my mother was organizing drawers, setting more clothes on hangers as my father sat on the edge of his bed. He looked up at us when we entered, nearly smiling as we walked towards him for a hug.

"Hi, Ma," we said, as she kept working silently. Nicole spotted a small machine by his bedside and asked my mother what it was.

"Oh, the nurse said to me this morning that daddy has sleep apnea—"

"What's that?" asked Nicole, alarm sounding through her voice. I watched her slight face grow anxious.

"It's when he stops breathing for several seconds—so they put the oxygen on him when he sleeps so that when he stops breathing he still gets air." My mom looked at us and saw we were worried. "It's

OK—now they know another thing that is the matter. But maybe now he will sleep better," she told us.

Soon afterwards, we heard her small steps and heavy squeaks of her walker against the tile in the hallway. Adeline entered much like yesterday, quietly, studying us all once again.

"Tell your father this is NOT an outhouse!!" she yelled upon entering. "This is MY house!" she screamed, and suddenly looked at my sisters and me with her small, blue eyes I remembered well.

"OK, Adeline. I will tell him," my mother said as she looked at my sisters and me with a smirk. "Nicole, go call the nurse," she added quietly.

Patty soon came in, explaining, "Oh! I'm so sorry! She really doesn't mean it," and I realized this would come to be a pattern with our friend Adeline Kirby. "Come on, Adeline. I'll take you to your room." I watched Patty as she guided Adeline's walker towards the door. I could hear Adeline's whining, telling her over and over again that that was indeed her house. And surely it wasn't an outhouse, at that.

We all left his room shortly after and took seats among the patients in the common area. The sun shone brightly through the windows, as the curtains were pulled back. We were eye-level with the cars that drove through the roundabout, the cars that stood waiting for their passengers, loved ones saying goodbye to their grandmothers, and grandfathers being walked to their families. I saw a few young people walk quickly up the path. They were holding green aprons and smocks, their uniforms hanging loosely in their tired arms and hands. I studied their faces, unassuming and young, and I figured I would soon come to know them well enough.

"Hello! Do you live here?" I turned to face a gray-haired woman with big wire-framed glasses and kind eyes. She had caught me off guard. I wondered if she was like Wilma, who chose to stay within those walls.

"Hi. What's your name?" I asked her, motioning to Flavia to come and meet her with me.

"I'm Evelyn. What's your name?" she asked, moving her head up and down as she enunciated each word.

"Stefania—and this is my sister, Flavia," I told her.

"Oh! S-s-fana. Fab—What strange names!" she said, then quickly pointed to my sister's shirt. "Oh! My son went to the University of . . . Kennedy."

Flavia smiled and glanced at me as we both quickly looked down at her shirt that read "University of Kentucky."

"Really?" Flavia said, and then began laughing. "That is wonderful." Soon after, we took a seat closer to our parents.

"Operator!! Operator!" screamed Cleda, who was still seated in her armchair against the wall.

"Alright, Cleda. That's enough," Patty yelled from across the room. "Like I said, she used to be a phone operator. She likes to call us Operator to get our attention."

"Really? How old is she?" My mom asked.

"She's 103. Had her birthday not too long ago," Patty said, as she approached Cleda.

"Hello? What the hell do you want? Eh?" Cleda said loudly, squinting her eyes towards Patty.

"Oh, Cleda. Won't you be a little nicer?" asked Patty.

"Oh, you're a doll, sweetie. Hey! HEY! Operator, can you get me a drink?" Cleda asked suddenly.

We must have sat in the common room for a few hours. Every now and then, a new name and face would enter our lives and we'd spend a moment or so getting acquainted. My father mainly sat at a table, chuckling or sitting still, not moving. We were exploring and trying to find a way to find comfort in the strange air we now shared with the others around us who decorated the pale white walls of the unit. And we found ways to laugh—ways to stop and pause without running—and ways to finally exhale.

A FEW WEEKS passed, and my father remained. At first Nicole and I would ask my mother sparingly if we were taking him home. Flavia would become angered at our prodding. Working full-time and in a long-distance relationship (her boyfriend still had one year left at the University of Illinois) put a further strain on her. I always felt guilty living away from home, missing most of the nights she and my mother would fight about my father—missing most of the nights when Nicole would be screaming at the both of them to stop. I missed most of the final nights they'd take turns putting him to bed, taking off his socks, like I had those nights he'd come home from work. They'd undress him and put him in his pajamas, maybe try to brush his teeth. I missed most of the nights when he'd get up right as they left the room and start pacing again, and the routine of night would begin.

It was like having divorced parents who lived in separate homes—and I had to be sure to find a balance somehow. It was difficult getting accustomed to the sights and sounds of that Alzheimer's Unit. Nicole and Flavia would tell me about new patients they'd meet, and share some funny stories about Cleda and Evelyn's latest quirky comment. When I'd come on weekends, we would all be there together.

My mother especially made her presence known. She voiced her concern whenever she found reason—and just to be sure his treatment was still adequate and remained constant and respectful when she wasn't around, she took a job working in dietary in February, about a month after his first night. She donned a green apron and met those young people I had seen outside. She became friendly with the other workers and knew almost everyone by their first name. My mother revolved her entire life around my father, and now she had added the nursing home. But it was for his dignity that she worked the hardest—if he lost everything else, his dignity was going to remain intact.

I WAS BEGINNING to feel the sense of habit settling about my sisters and me. This was going to be a new addition to our lives. For my sisters, they would go everyday nearly—but I was restricted to the weekends. And when I'd come alone or with just my mother, who came day after day, I'd stay behind after she'd leave. Or I'd come alone on a Saturday or a Sunday while she lay on the couch and tried to rest.

Alone, I didn't quite open up to everyone around me as quickly as my sisters or my mother did. I was still as cold as the windowpane in my father's room. And I seemed to put a space between me and the others for a bit longer than my family. I was still, of course, so angry, and it would take, yet again, the changing season to bring about the same change in me.

But that sense of habit settled more quickly than acceptance—that I know for certain.

Just like he did at home, he walked around and around, touching everything he could, and I would spend hours with him, just following him. I knew he probably wouldn't notice if I took a break, but my guilt over being away from him chained me to his every move.

One afternoon, as I followed my father, trying hard not to lead him, we approached Cleda. I watched his eyes grow round and airy, as he leaned in towards her, as she sat absentmindedly on a chair. He smiled, chuckling to himself. I soon realized he was trying to joke with her— tease her affectionately as I'd often see him do with children.

"What the hell are you doin'? What the hell do you want?" yelled Cleda, as my dad became even more amused glancing at me and down again at Cleda. She could sense his face inches away from hers—and though her cataract-embalmed eyes could hardly make out his face, she had a sense of who it was.

"He's only joking, Cleda. He doesn't mean to make you mad," I told her soothingly.

"Well, tell him to quit it! Always comin' around over here . . . doing God knows what!"

My dad frowned jokingly; he feigned offense. But he didn't hold a grudge, and he quickly tired of Cleda and shuffled onwards. Most of the women would sit for hours in those chairs bordering the windows in the common room, just like Cleda. One would always hum, others sat nodding on and off, and still more would mumble to themselves. Evelyn always smiled at us as we walked by, her short gray hair shaking a bit as her head bobbed up and down. She had a scratchy, rustic laugh and lifelines adorning her face. Evelyn had become a regular face in the room, while Wilma usually sat apart from the others or sat inside her room during her bad days, when breathing was most difficult. I wouldn't get a chance to really know Wilma as I would have liked—save for the first moment I met her, the calming sensation she seemed to share.

I followed my father as he turned again onto the white tiled hallway, where all the rooms to the patients' bedrooms lay. I walked, he scuffled, and every so often he'd grab my hand. He'd reach for it purposefully—hold it in his own, gently, just as a father should. I didn't know exactly why he was doing it—and I battled within my mind over whether or not it was a tic or something involuntary that pushed him to hold my hand. I'd be able to push away any doubts though and just revel in the feelings that holding his hand gave me. I felt a happiness and nostalgia overcome me, weakening my step; I'd nearly falter under the weight of it.

At the end of the hallway, two doors on opposite sides stood ajar, and he led me inside. First, he'd walk towards the windows, fiddle with the blinds, touch the windowsills and walk towards the small nightstand. I'd grow tired standing, watching him, looking as though he were searching for something he'd lost. I didn't want him to think I was bored, so I'd fiddle with objects right alongside him. I'd ask him questions and point to things, and he'd shake his head. He looked so serious, reminiscent of the face I remember—him reading intently, pointing to sentences he'd find in books, ideas he'd read and try to share with me. Yet it felt excruciating to think about how he was back then, back when the eyes I was staring at now—along with his expression—mirrored his determination. I would try and see him only as he was now, restless and childlike, searching for something his dementia seemed to demand.

Eventually, he'd grow tired of the space he was exploring and walk slowly around, and I'd follow him to the room across the hall. This

room was more crowded with furniture and made me more appre-
hensive about letting him wander on his own. I tried to lead him so
he wouldn't fall, trip on chairs or hurt himself.

I never knew if he realized I was there beside him. I always sort of
hoped, instead.

And then one day, he was holding my hand as though he was five
again while we traveled down the hall. We entered into a room and
then he squeezed my hand tighter. I turned to look at him and our
eyes met. His own seemed so sure and steady and even happy. And
just as clearly as I remember the tile beneath our feet and the sunlight coming in through the curtains of the crowded room, he spoke.
Without a stutter or a moment of hesitation—without any sign that
he was sick, he quickly, clearly said, "You're my buddy."

I smiled at him and watched as he seemingly nodded his head
and then turned his eyes away from me. He again started touching
walls and doorknobs, paddling fitfully as he returned to his imag-
inary entranceways and paths and special rooms. My face grew
hot and my eyes swelled as I followed him, touching whatever he
touched, inspecting whatever he inspected. I followed his every
movement as I silently told him, "Daddy, I'll be your little girl
forever."

ON THAT SAME tiled hallway, my father and I would often find some
traffic. Depending on the hour, any number of those patients could
have been walking outside their rooms or back inside again. Pat was
one such woman we'd see most days. Pat had eyes that sometimes
sparkled—on a face that sometimes smiled in a childish way, as
though she were hiding a secret so pleasant she could barely keep it
in. She walked up and down the white corridor, on that slippery floor,
pushing her walker awkwardly in front of her. Hunching forward,
she tended to keep her left shoulder above the right.

As my father and I made our way back into the common area one
afternoon, just as lunch was being doled out from a woman dressed

as my mother was daily, in a green apron and a hairnet, we passed by Pat, who stood clenching her walker.

"Pat? Pat? It's time for lunch, Pat. Come on now, turn around," the nurses from the desk called to her, trying to get her to make that small walk back to her seat she shared with three other women. Pat ignored them; I think I even heard her mumble something back in protest.

I went towards her, leaving my father to walk towards his table by himself; I wanted the nurses to help the others who had been waiting patiently in the common room. I knew getting Pat to come around would take a minute or two.

"Pat?" I said as I made my way slowly towards her. And she stopped. Her pale pink slippers were planted firmly before her walker.

"Could you help me?" she asked me, smiling pleasantly.

She squinted and put her hand up to her mouth, trying to show me that I should be quiet. "I need to get out of here. Let's go." At that, she picked up her feet and pushed on that walker and stepped heavily away. I followed.

I laughed a little at her saying this and somehow made her smile back. "Pat, come on. Let's go eat. I think we're having chicken."

"Eat? Oh! Are they having chicken? I love chicken." She turned then and stepped aside to let me accompany her down the hall. I felt victorious. She was simply enchanting, like a little lamb, until she changed.

As we walked, looking at one another after every other couple of steps, she suddenly stopped. She began shaking with such anger as it climbed up further into her mind. It was the second version of Pat that came to me then.

"Where are we going? I need to get out of here! I'm gonna kill myself!!!" She began to cry, and I held her hand. She pushed it away and shook her head.

"Come on Pat. Let's go. Everything is OK." She still stood shaking her head at me spitefully while she wept. I imagine I felt her tears land at my feet while a second later she said, "OK," her tears freezing midway from falling.

We continued on to the common room and I felt proud of my efforts, and of Pat for finally agreeing to go eat. She sat at her table and I made my way to my father, who sat alone now, since Adeline had caused too many problems sitting with him—"Can I have your fruit? What is wrong with you? Can't you sit somewhere else?" she would say.

As I fed my father, I'd turn every now and then to glance at Pat. After just a few bites of her meal, her mood shifted once more. With her walker at her side, she sat with her head slammed against the tabletop, and her white fluff of hair sitting like marshmallows on her head. I could hear her crying.

EVENTUALLY, VISITS WERE no more than habits, and the road to the nursing home, the right turns and lefts, the stop lights and intersections, became instincts I'd follow without so much as a second wind to keep me going. And I know it was the same for each of us, my sisters and my mother. After a few weeks, we knew it was certain that he would never come home again. The nurses themselves would tell my mother how surprised they were that she kept him home for so long. It was a mark of pride for my mother to hear them tell her. She had done her best, and she was finally being recognized.

We came to see the Bethesda Meadows welcome sign, the perfectly planted trees and blooming flowers around the pavilion and sidewalk—I know we all began to see the sign with just as much anxiety as comfort, and with as much anger as love.

It surely must have been in the coming of spring on this particular day when my mother drove with me to visit my dad. We pulled in to the driveway and made what had then become our familiar walk up towards the nursing home on the stone walkway beneath the large pavilion. My mom motioned towards the first-floor windows.

"Look, Stefania. You can see the patients! Look, there's Evelyn!" She pointed as she motioned me to follow her towards the side of the building, in front of the windowpanes. There, we saw Evelyn walking around the tables, and farther inwards we could spot a few nurses feeding patients snacks and medicine.

"A few days ago, I was walking here, Stefa, and then I saw daddy. He was walking by the windows, looking at everything, touching things, and then he looked out the window and he saw me coming. I walked over to him and then his eyes opened wide and he tapped on the window glass, and he was smiling," my mother said, as she brought me closer to the spot where he had seen her. "I told him, 'I'm coming in now—go wait by the door, Giovann—'" She laughed, and I did as well. "He started to nod—like a little puppy dog. I told him, 'go wait by the door, and I pointed to the doorway by the nurses, and then he nodded again and walked away."

I imagined her speaking to him through the glass; I imagined his excitement at seeing her and her's for him having noticed. In my mind, I imagined her frowning for a minute, thinking to herself, "I'm coming . . ." touching the glass, letting it slide from her hand.

Chapter 21

My window in Zio Marco's car must have been cloudy from the dirt and dust of the hours of driving. Whenever he rents a car to pick us up it is almost always air-conditioned, so for the most part, we sit snugly, breezy and cool. But like many Italians, because the price of gas is so high, he often opts out of using the air and instead relies on the wind from outside to cool him down.

On that day, the only discomfort I felt sat beside my foot and inside my heart as his urn sat for the last time beside me.

Our ride was mostly silent, and any conversations we had passed by unremembered, sweeping up and out the window. I wondered how Nicole and Flavia were as they got closer—were they still singing together like they always did when Flavia would come home from Italy? She'd bring home a CD from an Italian band or a singer that she'd know we'd love and play it over and over again until my mother would start to love it and take it in her car as well. "Where the hell did my CD go?" she'd ask, sitting in her driver's seat, realizing the CD player was empty. "Mom should really start asking first—" Flavia would say, before she'd start to change the radio channels, second after second with her right hand sitting still over the seek buttons and her other hand resting solidly on the wheel.

Nicole and I would look over at each other, getting annoyed at the way Flavia would skip over songs after just seconds. "I get paranoid that something better is on," she'd tell us, and Nicole would say, "Oh yeah, Fla?"

On weekends when my mother would work early and the three of us would find ourselves all at home, Flavia would drive us to the nursing home. It was on one of these sisterly outings that she took out her latest Italian find and put it in the CD player. She and Nicole were already familiar with him—he had a slow song that would put us all in the mood for singing even if singing was the last thing we wanted to do.

Once we started reversing down the driveway, Flavia raised the volume of their favorite song.

"Come on, Stef! Sing along!!" Flavia yelled to me, eyeing me through the rear view mirror. I sat quietly and smiled at her.

Flavia and Nicole suddenly started singing, more like yelling along, with Mauro DiMaggio.

"You do not belong here—you jump off the sand whale—and now that you feel, god's godda be had!" They yelled in unison, falling back into their seats, laughing.

"Uhh—what the hell was that??!" I asked, suddenly interested.

"That's his English solo! Why? Does it not make any sense?" Flavia asked, smirking, lifting one eyebrow above the other and playing it again.

THERE WERE TIMES I'd blast the music so loudly in my dorm room—loud and booming beats of Nine Inch Nails or Korn—music I would listen to in the car rides with Claudio, or Claudia and in my past summers going to Pacentro. But on one evening, I sat alone at a coffee shop with my head bent over my tattered gray notebook in which I would write poems, feelings, thoughts to do with college, my mind, my father, his mind and my family.

In this tattered notebook, I wrote down dialogue, quotes, and snippets of every day I lived that needed a bit more time to relive. And it was here that I wrote down the moment I sat and listened to soothing and much calmer music—simply Tori Amos and just her voice playing against the backdrop of what I started feeling the minute she said the word "Daddy," and I stopped what I was doing.

I tore away the page on which I was writing something else and started to write anew. She continued on with her song, singing

"Father," and I felt, suddenly, the familiar pain in my heart, the sharpness of it, the sudden surge of blood running into my chest; my breath became shallow. And it was as though the well behind my eyes I kept up while away at school began to bleed, as the cuts and scars atop my legs and my arms suddenly throbbed. I listened to her sing the line that I remember hearing so many times before—"When you gonna love you as much as I do?" According to my words in my notebook, it was as though I felt she were fading into him as he'd shake me again, looking at me, pleading with me to stop. I remember him asking me that same question so many times—my father grabbing my shoulders in agony, teary edged and pleading with me to stop—to let go and love myself.

She continued: "Cause things are gonna change," she said, and I knew it wouldn't be for the better. "Things change" I heard, as I sat with my head in my hands and tried not to bring about too much attention.

I was overwhelmed after hearing that song. I got up to leave; throwing everything in my bag, I walked out as fast as I could and cried. It felt as though she were taunting me in a way—Tori Amos singing me a song that would reduce my whole life into just scenes upon scenes of my hardest times. Making me realize I never did stop. That I never really ever stopped to love myself as much as he did. At least not until it was too late and he was gone.

So with that guilt I had inside of me—that guilt I didn't really know existed until the lighting was just so and a song would play and my mind was listening—I finally let a layer of myself feel something other than anger for the first time. I was beginning to let go of anger and starting, instead, to grasp onto grief, to regret. It was during those several months in that nursing home that I finally decided I was not angry—guiltily, I was only sad.

I CRIED A lot by myself at college and again in the car, driving to the nursing home on weekends when I'd go alone. One afternoon,

I came to him as he walked up and down the hallway in the Alzheimer's unit shuffling his feet, his left side now turning more and more powerless, dragged by his stronger right side. It showed the progression of the destruction of his brain. And I followed him like I did before, like I had done over and over again, past the same old worn faces of the grandmothers and grandfathers in the common area, past the nurses laughing and joking to one another and to patients as they handed them their drugs, the tokens of their sickness. I imagined those pills as just tranquilizers and candy canes, just medicine and treats every few hours or so to calm them down and be more malleable.

After his medicine, after the tranquilizing effects settled in, he became again a sleepy man, a calmer man, but less a man than a voided body of a man.

I followed him into his room, as it was time again for a nap. I often tried to lay him down after his medicine. At least in the nursing home, it seemed to work much better than it had at home. I wonder if the pills were just stronger or if the routine was more appealing to the effects of sleep.

"Come here, daddy. Let's lie down a little," I said as I laid him down onto his hospital bed, lowering the bars down on either side. I adjusted his pillow, removed his slippers like I had done years before, though when I then removed his slippers in the nursing home that night, I couldn't remove his socks—his geriatric socks I found sticking tightly around his legs. To help with circulation. I often saw these thick tan-colored stockings on the women walking with their walkers, on Pat with the mood swings and the gentle smile, and on Adeline, who was growing sicker, skinnier and quieter.

But my father, he was wearing them now around his tan skin, his black leg hair crushed beneath its tightness. I paused a moment to look at him as he lay there atop his white, starched pillow. He looked straight above while every so often closing his eyes, and then I raised the sheet over him. Sitting a moment on a chair to see if he would sleep, I soon heard his snoring

How it used to bother Flavia those days we traveled. Disney world, beaches, island escapes and ferry rides—how I wish I didn't waste so many years in between the times when I would laugh with him, begging him to join me in the sun and water—to the days when I'd sit in the shade, trying desperately to keep pale and frail.

I remember Flavia complaining in our hotel room those nights before Nicole was born. As Flavia lay beside me in a queen-size bed, she'd call to my dad, who lay sleeping in the bed next to ours. She'd yell his name out until he'd wake suddenly, choking on a last inhalation. I pretended it didn't bother me. I'd go so far as to complain to Flavia that she was keeping *me* awake—and yell at her to leave daddy alone. "It's not that annoying!" I'd say.

Of course, I did have trouble sleeping through it too. But then I wouldn't have been his buddy, would I, if I had done what Flavia had done? And even what my mother often did as well—calling out his name just before he'd fall asleep entirely.

I stared at my father as he slept on his hospital bed, the snoring stronger than it was minutes before, a tell-tale sign he was now asleep. The pauses between his breaths unnerved me, but now that I knew it was the sleep apnea, I let the anxiety run its course over my back, down my spine, dissolving somewhere at its base. I got up from the chair I had set beside him, watching him fall deeper and deeper into sleep. I didn't realize then, but it was as if I were watching a patient sleep, a child sleep, as though he were afraid of the dark and I had kept guard for him, promising him I would not leave.

I never had that fear as a child— the fear of the dark. I never used it as an excuse for my parents to come to my room at night. No, I wanted a different reason behind his visits and my mother's when they'd come to me in my bedroom. What I wanted most of all from them was to be read to. And I loved the different ways my mother and my father sounded as they read over the words in my books. I loved the way my mother's heavy accent rolled the r's and lengthened the e's, made the i's much more like e's and the e's like a's. And I loved her cadence, the music of her sentences rising and falling, like the ways she'd speak to my father in Italian.

My father, instead, would read to me quite calmly, quite lightly, and I could almost still hear his accent and feel his arms against mine as we'd try in vain to fit in the small spaces of my own twin bed. His voice was never too daring, too deep or too light. It was my father's nighttime story voice and I can still sense its outlines now. But the truth is, I can't recall its timbre, its pitch—I can only remember the way I felt. And the feeling has fleshed out the sounds and made a memory of only its echo.

I SAT DOWN beside him, making sure to sit lightly, because I knew how hard it would be to lay him down again. I took off my left shoe, then my right, held onto the rim of the bed, knocking my heels against the metal bars. Then I lay down, my head beneath his, parallel to his shoulders. I felt small again; I felt the way I used to feel, as the memory came to me of mornings in my parents' room. Or times when I would cry again and again for things I may have done not knowing it was my guilt, my second self, the one who had since lain dormant and who was now breaching the waters for air.

I looked up to him, to his chin hanging lax above me and down to his arms. One lay over his stomach and his other lay by his side. I slipped that arm over me as I stealthily tried to share my father's twin bed.

And then I laid my arm around his stomach, resting my hand atop his own. And I held him, tightly, and suddenly—suddenly, I couldn't remain quiet and calm. I couldn't just watch him, just hold him, just hug him. I cried and dug my face into his side, my tears leaving puddles on his arm. I let go a few words of my anger and my sadness, mumbling them into his arm, into his belly. As I cried harder I grasped him tighter, and I imagined god and I thought of religion and thought of blaming hope and blaming life and hating all of them together. And I cried, trying to get myself as close to him as possible, holding him as tightly as I could without waking him, imagining he was holding me too. Imagining he was telling me, "Don't worry, Stefania. Things are gonna change—I love you." And then I shut my eyes and calmed myself down, breathing steadier, breathing deeper—my tears falling slower. My fears melting into sleep.

I DON'T RECALL how long we stayed like that. I do remember the drool I felt from my mouth sticking to my cheek. And how long did I stay after he awoke? He must have just stood up along with me and either made his way to the common area or veered left out his door and towards the end of the hall.

Evelyn lived down at that end. And she was often found in her room during the middle of the day—she wasn't one for sitting still in one of the chairs that lined the windows, listening to Cleda's "Operator!" or Pat's manic laughter.

Evelyn would try to talk to my father. "Hello there! How are you doing today?" she'd say, and normally he would keep on walking, ignoring her or any one else, though I'm sure he just must not have noticed. The something pressing in his mind was always much louder than anything else.

Evelyn would turn to me then. "Hello, would you like to see my house?" she asked me.

I left him as he made his way into one of the abandoned rooms at the end of the hall, and I went into Evelyn's home.

"See this? This is my chair—my favorite chair," she said as she planted herself proudly on a very homely brown lounge chair, adorned with a quilt. They added years and depth and such warmth to her cozy room filled with pictures of family and old-fashioned decor. She had many wooden trinkets and shapes and cats and frames, and it seemed to be a theme she kept—one of country and home sweet home. I got a sense of who she was when I stepped into her home, her nursing home bedroom—more than when I spoke with her.

She was a proud mother and had photos to prove it. I knew my own mother was proud as well—I hoped so, anyway. I hadn't offered her much during the years before—I hadn't made anything easier on her, except now I was changing. I was changing and she was noticing and my sisters did as well—the way I'd talk to them more and open up more. I would joke with them more as well, even about the patients and the workers with whom my mother became friends.

"Stef—how cute is Kevin?!" Nicole would ask—"I can't believe it—I just want to throw up when I see him!"

"Oh god, Nic—you mean 'Nursing home Ken'?" I said as we ate altogether once in the cafeteria, laughing as we coined a new nickname for a coworker of our mother's at Bethesda.

For we were a unit in ourselves the way we persevered, coming as one and then dispersing to mingle among the others who offered us distraction and solace while our father began losing his steps.

"Did you see, Stefa? He can't walk anymore—" my mother told me not too long before I had noticed it myself.

"What do you mean?" I had asked her. I didn't notice much—maybe yes, that he did walk slower, seemed to fumble more—to stumble. But it wasn't that big a deal, I thought.

"Stefania, it's his disease. It's starting to progress more. Pretty soon, he's going to have to switch floors," she told me, without any change in her voice. It was a simple fact she was relating to me. She was telling me so I'd be ready. In the same way that she had "told" me years before the morning after she caught me drinking in my room. Only this time—it was different. She wasn't trying to hurt me with facts that were going to happen *one day.* She wasn't trying to shake sense into me like she had that morning when she used the only thing she thought would reach me. My mother was now telling me so I would know and be aware like she was. Because I didn't need reaching anymore.

"The fourth floor—that's where they go. The ones who can't walk. They all have wheelchairs," she said, and I imagine myself inside the cafeteria then, looking at my mother as she stands in a green apron and a hairnet.

I see her smile as she says, "Hello Aldrin! Hi Sarah! Did you meet my daughter?" while she takes change from a customer paying for their hot meal or a salad.

I stand before her and then walk towards the tables set in front of her. Long tables like they had in high school, in middle school and elementary. Those tables that would sometimes act as socializing centers, craft centers. If I think hard, I almost see the outlines of a school-sponsored sale of gifts for Mother's Day, Christmas and Father's Day. And if I squint I can see myself picking up a small keychain with miniature flathead screwdrivers: one red, one green, one yellow. I see myself giving it to him on Christmas and him studying it intently before my mind wanders and I see the flowers he'd set on the fireplace hearth. For on Mother's Day, my father would go to Sam's Club and buy roses and set them out in vases. He'd get beautiful bouquets for each of his girls and for his wife for whom he'd also buy a card always signing it with something sweet and ending with something like, "from your amazing, adoring husband." He'd write, "I love you."

And on Father's Day, Flavia, Nicole and I would be expected to give him a small gift or a card. Nicole would draw a picture or make something at school. She was always so crafty, and still is—her artistry coming in handy especially when money seems a bit scarce. I can imagine Flavia driving up to the grocery store we lived near to buy a last-minute card and a balloon she'd put in the kitchen beside the card that she'd sign, "I love you."

I remember writing him a poem one year for both his birthday and Father's Day. It rhymed—the poem—and it was very colorful. I drew a turtle on it, my trademark, and handed it to him proudly. For me, writing a poem was easy to do, and for him it was the dearest gesture, just as it was for my mother on Mother's Day.

And in the nursing home, the nurses didn't take a break on Father's Day, although they didn't completely ignore the day, either. It seemed to have an even stronger presence there, with signs and balloons and a special meal for the patients who were lucid on other floors. It came and it settled snuggly on June 15, 2003, five months after the first night we brought him there.

I walked into the Alzheimer's unit, and noticed the sign first—"Happy Father's Day"—that hung above the nurses' station.

"Hi, Stefania!" Nurse Patty rang out to me as I smiled warmly at her and looked around. The man and woman who held hands as they sat in their separate recliners were most likely in their rooms. I had discovered that the man's name was Buck and he was married with children. His wife visited him and he didn't know who she was. Instead, he'd hold onto his fellow patient's hand, squeezing it daily and believing she was his wife. It was heartbreaking to know that Buck's wife was there and knew how he had replaced her. But she understood. Every member of every family of every patient there understood. We kept going though, kept walking forward and moving despite the pain that we found in that unit.

And I kept walking, searching for my father among the others on that special day—on that very special Father's Day.

I found him wandering like he always was, before Nurse Patty yelled out, "John! John, your daughter's here!" He did recognize his name and he'd stop or look around or move his eyes towards his name. That day he was in a polo tee shirt and sweatpants. He was in a good mood—giggling and walking for the most part without dragging his leg. At least I didn't notice much of a struggle as he walked, because I was too busy memorizing his smile.

The nurses wanted to take our picture to put behind the station on the corkboard where other pictures were taped up and thumb-tacked in.

"Here, we have one for all the fathers. Put it on your dad—we'll take a picture!" one of the nurses said as she handed me a boutonnière to pin on his shirt.

"Daddy—Dad, stand still," I told him as he became more and more restless. They placed a sombrero on his head and he smiled even more—laughing with us as we all felt a breeze of normalcy sweep through. In the strangest way, seeing him in a silly sombrero was the most normal way I'd seen him in a long time.

In the picture they took, I look directly into the camera and smile awkwardly as my fingers try to pin the flower into the front of my father's shirt.

He stands bent a bit forwards, amused and seemingly about to speak. His eyes had begun to travel like his feet did, slower and uneven. His eyes didn't keep a steady stare and one eye was lazier than the other.

We are both glazed with a bit of sweat from the heat outside because perhaps we had also come in from a walk that Father's Day afternoon.

So when my mother told me about his disease progressing, I didn't feel the panic rising like I used to. I felt another layer of mourning, mainly, for the steps I would soon stop hearing coming down the hall, up the hall and back down again.

Chapter 22

The decision to move my father upstairs came rather quickly, I thought. I think there was in fact a date set for when he would leave because I remember sitting on the green vinyl sofa chair, looking at all the patients and trying my best to remember every detail. Every detail that I felt was important and special I wrote later in my notebook, knowing I would one day try to meet them all again in writing.

"Honey—where's the rest of your dress?" Cleda yelled to Flavia one hot summer day.

"It's my dress—it's how it's supposed to look, Cleda!" Flavia said walking up to her, shouting somewhat so she'd hear. She stood before Cleda, in her tanned skin and halter-top, with her hair swept up away from her slight face.

"Well, that ain't no dress—" Cleda responded with utter dismay on her face, her mouth sunken inwards and pinched together.

And then Evelyn would walk by, laughing to herself as the gray in her hair shone brilliantly beneath the lights above us.

"My teeth! Where's my teeth?!" Cleda would soon yell as Nurse Patty and the rest would laugh and I would chuckle softly, hearing Nicole's seal-like laughter matching my mother's as my father stumbled onwards. It was like that, the Alzheimer's Unit—moments of laughter and rest as my sisters, mother and I would listen to the patients, watching them and prodding them for more.

"Pat, you look so beautiful today," Nicole told her once, expecting her to smile back in return.

"I need to get outta here," Pat replied as her face began to tremble.

We learned to go along with the motions, learned to understand their idiosyncrasies. We went along with the rises and the falls, learning to see past the words and the moments, the hours spent as they'd stare or sit, some holding hands and others crying, some screaming while others laughed. We learned to imagine them well, to remember them before, floating as they were on the surface of the ever-changing waters of their illness.

I TALKED A lot about the patients to Dan and Jessie, filling our card games and chess games with glimpses of the women in the Alzheimer's Unit.

"You should've heard her—" I'd start to tell them, taking time out to light a cigarette.

But the talk would shift as they'd ask about my father.

"My mom says he's going to be moving upstairs soon. To the fourth floor," I told them one evening in September. "It's the floor that everyone goes when they can't walk anymore. When they're in the last stages . . . " and as my voice trailed off Jessie said, "I'm so sorry, Stefania."

Dan kept mostly silent, letting me talk or cry without judgment or pause. I could tell in the way he'd pull out another cigarette or watch his coffee mug sitting untouched and growing cold that he didn't know what to say. But he knew that he needed to listen and just show me that he was there for me and would continue to be no matter where this disease was going to take us.

Dan had, at that time, already been home about six months after leaving Florida his second semester of college. He had had a drunken night, and cut his hand after dramatically displaying a note for his friends to see on a door. He was depressed that evening and wanted to tell his friends and apologize for his odd behavior so he decided the most sensible way would be to hang up the note with a knife on a metal door. Dan's hand slid across the blade and severed his tendons. He had gotten surgery in the winter to fix the damage while battling speculation that he had instead tried to kill himself. Dan had spent his recovery mainly on the couch in his family's guest room, watching reruns of his favorite show, *Charmed*, and playing with his cats, Rudy and Max.

As I looked at Dan, his eyes heavy as usual from lack of sleep and too much smoking, his fingers on his damaged hand bent and still aching with scarring, I wanted to leave The Grind and drive. Jessie of course would come—she had been a necessary addition to our group as Dan and I became more and more similar. She added a touch of optimism and sunlight to our misty, smoke-filled car. I wanted to hang my hand out the window, gliding it through the air to the rhythm of whatever music would be playing, listening to Dan singing and Jessie speaking and nothing else.

But The Grind is where we stayed that night I told them he was growing worse, moving down another level in his demise, edging closer to the day he'd forget to smile.

After some silence, Dan said, "my dad is going to drive me to Columbia this weekend to start moving in."

"Oh my god! I still can't believe you were able to get that apartment upstairs," I said. I had signed a lease to live with Meagan my second year at school. It was a house on College Ave, split into apartments, and we felt lucky enough to get a small two-bedroom with a large kitchen in the basement. We didn't seem to care much yet about the fact that we had little sunlight and that our windows would barely serve to connect us with the sky. We were just excited to be living in our own apartment, creating a home and a refuge. We went a week ahead of classes to decorate our new place.

From morning until night, Meagan and I scrutinized every place-ment of picture frame and decorative stone. We made our way from one end to the other gradually and didn't stop until we were satisfied with every corner, every wall and every room. Meagan was an artist. She drew and painted, sang and wrote, and so together we tried to make a haven of sorts to match our every artistic whim. The kitchen was adorned with postcards of feminist quotes of women from the fifties, our bathroom was color-coordinated in greens and browns, *earthy tones*, and our wall in the living area was adorned with a piece of cloth surrounded by brightly colored painted coasters.

My room kept the facade of my teenage years: the dark posters with my favorite singer, Trent Reznor from Nine Inch Nails, black sheets and African masks. I added touches with candles and had bought a red velvet chair for no reason but its color, to enhance the dramatic effect of my room. I had a tapestry with purples and blacks that my mother had bought for me as well as a Dali poster, "Reflections of an Elephant," beside my bed. It was everything I felt and admired and needed at a time when I seemed to be losing a grip on everything else. This was the *first* time I had the chance to really make a space my own.

I grappled with where to place my black desk I had purchased at Goodwill a month before. I needed it in a prime location, I had thought, where I could sit and write without distraction and in perfect balance with space and distance from the door. Since I had no window, I could easily factor out distraction from the outside, though I would have welcomed it. Not having a window proved much more distracting than not. Sleep overcame me at any hour of the day and my seclusion in my room would be almost intoxicating—where there'd be nothing save for the images of elephants and Trent Reznor to stare at.

I kept my gray notebook on that desk, beside the pictures of my father and mother. My mother's is a bit out of focus as she sits on a ledge in front of the Monte Morrone, somewhere up the mountain towards Fonte Romana or the horses my father once ran to. She's dressed in a black shirt and bell-bottomed jeans and her hair is cut short, though I can tell it had been growing out for some time. The picture of her was taken not long after her mother died of cancer when my mother was sixteen. She's smiling from the point of view of where I can see, though through the blur of distance and poor focus, I can't quite grasp the look in her eyes.

In the picture of my father, he sits wearing a white baseball cap—it reads "Hawaii" in red. He's in a blue short-sleeved shirt and it brings out his summer tan and the brown glow of his eyes that look into mine with ease and peace. It must have been taken years ago, back when I was younger than Nicole, probably even before she was born, when I was five, maybe, or just turning six. It's the quiet I feel when I see it and the love I feel when I look at him that makes me write of it as though I'm looking at it now. It is emblazoned on my eyes even when I sleep at times.

Dan moved into a one-bedroom apartment right above Meagan and me. His living room was atop my bedroom, and every day I'd hear him laughing at a show he loved, hear his footsteps and the sudden creaking of the ceiling as he'd fall into his sofa. At times, I'd take a broom and chase him around, have a contest to see who would give up first—me with banging the broom on the ceiling or him stomping on the floor with his foot. I had to stop the game after dents started populating the ceiling and I feared more the labor it would take to fix it than to let Dan win.

"Stefania, you have to meet Irma though. She lives up there," my mother said as she made her way towards me, sitting at an empty table.

"Who is she?" I asked, wondering how in the world another woman could enter my life, another patient from Bethesda—how could another one really matter, really?

"Oh, Stefania, just wait," she said, and I nodded.

Chapter 23

Beneath the trees we drove, Zio Marco keeping speed, my mother keeping watch through her window. She had grown a bit more silent, though maybe it is just in my imagination. Perhaps I look back now and place my own emotions on her, the ones I feel as I emerge myself once more into the girl who sits quietly behind her uncle. The girl who now presses her foot against her father's urn more firmly than before, because beneath the trees they drive and soon the road widens just enough that only the sun now bears against her skin.

And it is there—through the window, I see it. Coming into focus more and more. Pacentro—standing cool and still in gray stone up above me. We follow it now, upwards, and I lean backwards, inert. I swallow back fear and resistance just as I had nearly a year before, and slowly my thoughts grow vivid, remembering and imagining, as though heavy as a mist, parted slowly with the shadowy outline of my father. The car shifted and I looked out the window as we turned, ascending.

As THE ELEVATOR doors opened, my eyes were instantly drawn to the August sun shining in through the sealed windows. To the side of the windows, back against the wall, was a large fish tank that must have been a source of pleasant distraction for the patients and the nurses up there on the fourth floor.

I saw him before anyone else came into focus. He was in a corner of the common area set against a wall with a framed picture hanging above him. From what I can recall, it was perhaps a flower—a pink flower with stem and leaves—though I could very well have imprinted my own image upon that very canvas.

He sat wretchedly hitting his hands against the tray, hearing the sounds and feeling the slight pangs but continuing, experimenting with his new power to inflict pain and produce sound.

My feet felt heavy against the tile and my heart caught in my throat—I could have fallen there amid the patients I now noticed, all in wheelchairs, many oblivious to anything around them, all invalid, all dying. I didn't give a face to any of them, just saw their broken bodies and made my way through the open spaces towards him.

And he didn't even look at me from across the room. He had for several months been losing the ability to focus both his eyes on me. He'd look at me for a few seconds but then turn his face away. And always, I could tell the way he looked at me was different than it ever was before. It was the same for all of us. We had grown used to it—thought it even normal now for him to avert his gaze from us as we tried to will him closer. So with his eyes that didn't look at me, and his feet that couldn't be trusted to not let out from beneath him—my father sat trapped in that large gray chair with the plastic tray locked in place.

I stood in front of him and I let the images settle, compacting like white snow before the road licks its sides. I tried to remember every detail. Knowing there would be many more days and months I'd spend at his side, I didn't overwhelm myself with the mental notes and strokes of capturing these images later. The fact that it was the first time I was seeing him confined like that was enough of a memory for the moment. It was the realization that this was where he had ended up—that this was my father, my faded hero, trapped and bleating in his geriatrics chair in the corner of the fourth floor.

As I made my way towards him, trying to ignore everything else around me, I would have passed by a woman tearing paper, sitting by herself in a flowered sunhat with her long, white hair cascading over her shoulders. I would have passed by her tablemate, who sat frowning, her hair gray and wavy, her nose sharp, her eyes dark. I would have passed another table, passed a woman who would later start crying, start shaking and start screaming. Her face was nothing but wrinkles and burrowed eyes inside her small face.

I would have passed a woman looking friendly who would glance at me before making her way to her room—walking, standing straight. Looking well. She'd soon shut her door, I know, opening it again, shutting it still.

Finally, I'd be just steps away and see in the corner of my eye a man, trembling and spitting, sitting by himself. He'd look up at me and I'd see a pair of watery blue eyes, kind eyes, and the only steady part of himself.

And my father, sitting beneath that framed forgotten picture. To his left and right, grand windows showing trees and far-off neighborhoods with mothers and fathers I would imagine sometimes—sitting happily around their kitchen tables—eating, laughing and loving. I looked at him, as he sat, and began with my own questions. I had started to ask him, "Daddy? It's me. How are you feeling? Are you hungry? Do you love me? Do you see me?" I hear myself ask as the image of myself blending into the movements of the car, into the angle of our ascent pushing me backwards into the seat and farther backwards to the very first day I went to visit him alone on the fourth floor.

THE FIRST TIME I walked towards the building knowing I would not be visiting him in the familiar Alzheimer's Unit on the first floor, I passed the window where not too long before I would have seen my father. He would have been walking around and around, zigzagging and weaving through the women who would have grown annoyed and angry. "Tell 'im to get the hell away from me!" Cleda would yell, toothless. And maybe my father would then pass the chair where Buck used to sit, grasping the hand of his substitute wife.

I walked without stopping to notice whether or not I'd see anyone I knew—keeping my head forward and my persistence solid. It was difficult making my way to the elevators. I almost turned after the front desk—before willing my feet to move simply forward.

It didn't take long to reach the floor, to wait for the doors to open and see the fish tank and perhaps a nurse standing at the moving cart preparing medicine for the patients on the floor. The nurses didn't look up at me, nor did anyone at the desk move to say hello. Not like downstairs, with Nurse Patty's throaty laughter filling up the silent spaces of fear every time I'd enter.

Up there on the fourth floor, the common area had no couches—just tables and chairs and wheelchairs. A TV was stationed in the front of the room, though no one really watched it besides the nurse's aides who walked back and forth in their scrubs. I remember there was one male nurse's aide who was skinny and pale, and I was instantly unnerved by him, fearing he'd look at me the way men at times look at women. I would have called him on it and hated him instantly had I caught him. I would have told my dad and he would have chased him down the hall and out the door, yelling at him to stay away from me. He would have protected me before returning to his room. With just a simple glance in my direction that aide flooded my mind with these scenarios that left me feeling sodden and semi-fatherless as I walked into my father's room that afternoon for the first time by myself.

What I saw—I never would have even considered a possibility. Downstairs, my father had had his own room, had had plenty of chairs for us when we visited, a TV my mom had bought just for him should he ever sit still to watch it. He had had a glass display panel outside his door, with our pictures in it and plenty of him as well and strong—in all shades and colors of sun and shade and age. The display seemed inviting and it reminded everyone who dared to forget that once, not too long ago, his forgetting never seemed such a threat.

There was a man lying on a twin bed in my father's new room and all I could smell was him. The stench was sour and pungent with sharp edges and he glanced at me and I at him, expressionless and empty. He wore a white A-line shirt, in my memory, and blue shorts—but this could all just be made up. He could've also been eating a greasy sandwich from one hand and in the other, a remote control. A smuggled in beer beside his elbow on the small bedside table and a gold chain hanging from his neck would be the other touches I could add to this picture. But these again are just brush strokes against his empty sketch because all that's left painted is the corner where my father lay on a mattress set against the wall on the floor.

I quickly went to him as I saw him struggling and squirming. He was sweaty and mumbling and his face was bright red. I panicked and held onto his arms and tried to reach him still—"Daddy—daddy, I'm sorry. Why are you so hot? Are you OK? Dad? Hang on, I'll get a nurse," I started saying until I moved the sheet away from his legs which had gotten twisted up together and found him without a diaper—without anything on at all.

I was enraged. I thought, "What the hell is going on here!? Where the fuck is his diaper? His shorts! And he's on the floor and it smells and it's fucking hot!" I went outside, leaving without telling him, knowing it probably wouldn't have made a difference. I passed by the nurse's aide and looked at him quickly, contemplating whether I should tell him or not. I decided to tell the nurses.

"Um, my father—he's John Silvestri. He has *nothing* on—his pants—he has no diaper on!" I managed to say, as tears welled in my eyes. I didn't want to cry. I wanted to maintain control and take care of him. I wanted to get the situation fixed as soon as possible and I didn't want to appear weak. I wanted to be like my mother, who I had seen time and again, yelling in her accented voice at nurses, administrators—for one thing or another. Making a scene whenever she felt threatened or felt my father's dignity was on the line.

"Yes, we are aware. We do that to the patients every now and then. Let them air out. It helps with skin irritation from the diapers," one nurse told me. Her hair was cut short and hairsprayed in all directions. Her nails were well manicured. She pinched her eyebrows together and looked at me pityingly, I thought.

"But I don't understand! He's red and he's sweating! His mattress is on the floor—" I continued, still seething and close to tears.

"Your father was very agitated. We put his mattress down to prevent him from falling off the bed," she continued—always with an answer for everything. "Please wait out here, we'll get your father dressed," the nurse said, as she and a nurse's aide walked coolly towards his door. I remained there, standing still. I didn't know what to do or say or feel. I felt ashamed for thinking that the nurses didn't know—for assuming they may have ignored him—leaving him nearly naked, seemingly cowering in the corner. I stood and waited. I watched the other nurses administer medicine to mute patients and felt ill at ease in my new environment. It was so big up there—so alien. I didn't recognize a soul, save for my father—and he I hardly recognized at all.

I started to make my way towards the elevators, back towards the fish tank to stand. A woman sat on a bench, looking as though she may have been contemplating something. I wish I could conjure the details of her mouth and her eyes, of her shoes or her hands, but I can't. I feel her presence there and the window blinds I nearly hear, imagining them swaying slightly. I do recall the nurse calling for me again and me making my way towards my father's room where he sat in his geriatrics chair, his diaper on, his face returning to a simple tan. He didn't say a word as I whispered to him, "Do you feel better, dad? I'm so sorry you were so hot before." I pushed his chair out of his room and back towards the common room, towards his other corner.

As we sat, I stared at him. I had begun trying to memorize every detail of my father. His hands—I needed to make sure those hands were inscribed on my eyes, on my heart. I often put his hand in mine and pushed his fingers down, making it feel as if he were holding it. The way we used to—even downstairs for brief moments. He would never look at me even though I would try my hardest to will his eyes toward my own. I did have his fingers. His large, flat fingernails. That's why my cousin Mario and I had similar hands when I was young—my hands come from my father's side. My hands come from him.

When I let go of his hands, I'd move up to his wrists, to the bone that stuck out towards the base of his hands. On the inside of his left wrist, he had a long, jagged scar that protruded from the surface of his skin. I look at my wrist now and try to remember if it was on the left or the right of the artery; I was in fifth grade when he got it, that I do remember. He was holding me above the water in the ocean.

We had gone to Hawaii that summer in fifth grade with the Rallos. I was eleven and he, forty-five—just three years shy of his diagnosis.

As usual, I had begged him to play with me in the water—"Dad! Let's go snorkeling—come on!!" I yelled, prying him from the sand beneath a tree where he and my mother and the Rallos were sitting. There were towels strewn about among baskets filled with toys and extra clothes and food—and diapers for Sophia. Nicholas was yet to be born.

"OK, OK," he said, as he took off his sunglasses and hat, following me as I grasped onto our snorkeling gear.

"Do you want to use the flippers?" I asked him, hoping he'd say yes. We never used them and I wasn't confident that either one of us could even be able to wear them well, but they seemed fun, seemed different, and I was feeling daring, I suppose.

"No, let's get them later," he had said. I wonder if he didn't want me to see him struggle. But then I remember the way he stood to dive into the small waves that came to crash at his ankles. The way he bent his knees and put his arms together above his head and ahead of him to dive. And right as the small bend of water seemed almost at his waist, he dove, his back hardly submerged. Even my mother, sitting with a magazine against her bent knees, her sunglasses on her face, laughed at the sight of him as he rose first to his knees and then his feet, spitting up water from his mouth and nose; his thin hair he'd comb to the side, hanging straight down into his eyes.

Yes, those arms were funny, at times scary—at times, those arms were the one thing I needed for me to let go of anger, take a break from sadness. Those arms are the arms I spit on when he'd tried to help me, too. As I'd sit on his green recliner, my face contorted in miserable expressions, he'd try to talk to me—as my mother would try to coddle me. And I did nothing for those arms, except my own that I would later hurt and punish. Except by the time I sat and studied his own, I had stopped hurting myself. I didn't want to hurt them any longer.

Maybe that jagged scar on his wrist was the embodiment of all of my smaller scars rolled into one. All the suffering I would lay on myself, all held together on him. The scar sits now where a cyst had begun to hurt him and throb that day. After we had snorkeled, he had grasped me and thrown me in the air again and across the water until he cried out in pain. We had walked together to the hotel in search of ice, and the guilt that I had caused his pain stayed with me until I went to sleep that night, thinking it was all my fault. It seems I'd repeat this over and over again until I finally started to shed this guilty bondage to him and to her—to me still floating in the water on my own.

I PLANTED MY feet firmly on the floor beside him and rubbed his arm, looking at him all the while as he stared emptily ahead.

"Daddy? It's me. Do you see me? Do you love me? Daddy—are you cold? Are you warm?" I asked him. When he wouldn't answer, I began to tell him pieces of my college life—of course, only the parts I would have told him had he been well.

"I made the dean's list last semester, daddy. And Dan moved upstairs. I'm glad he's there, dad. He's helping me. Meagan and I have been living together. It's nice, our apartment. I've made good friends . . . "

Then, of course, I would not have told him about fighting with my mother—about Flavia and her checking my bank statements, yelling at me about money, about saving. And me selling blood plasma just so I could have more money to go out. It was Dan's idea, of course.

Those are the moments he can't take part in anymore, I'd think. And I'd think that perhaps if I told him, he might get upset. It all might shake him up and then how would he be?

My thoughts were interrupted by harshly creaking wheels. The sound came from behind me until it was beside me—slight scuffs of shoes against the tile interrupted by squeaks and skids.

I felt eyes staring at the back of me and smelled old youth driving towards me.

"Is that your father??" She pointed with her entire palm towards my dad, her fingers all crinkled together. She was dirty-mouthed and smelled though she was a bit more tame than my father's roommate. Hers was a smell less pointed, more musty than putrid.

I wrinkled my eyebrows towards her and nodded.

"Is that your father?" I figured she hadn't seen my head—like Cleda from downstairs, her blue eyes were cataract-embalmed beneath her large frames.

"Yes," I said.

"Who are you?" she asked me—blowing her stale, heavy breath in my direction. I turned towards her, thinking, "Why isn't she leaving me alone?"

I didn't want her near me. And instantly, I wanted to shield my father from her. I still felt nervous that these women might make him depressed and make him realize where he was. I never thought he was like any of them—and that white haired woman with the drooping mouth and small eyes surely was too much to handle at that moment.

"I'm Stefania," I did finally repeat.

But instead of turning away, she simply sat and stared at me—though she missed my face by inches. Her head seemed heavy as she tried again to meet my gaze.

After a second or so, she put her awkward sallow hands back into her lap and leaned forward towards me. Her breath was hot and smelled of spoiled milk. I cringed.

"Lavagna?" she asked me, her voice coming out squeaky and deep. Maybe she smoked when she was younger. I grew anxious that she would be my fate.

As she moved her arm again towards her head and wiped a bit of brownie into her gray hair, she squinted and began breathing loudly and heavily.

"No, Stefania—S-T-E-F-A-N-I-A," I said loudly, then turned my chair against her and ended our first meeting.

She seemed satisfied with my response and rolled away, pushing on the ground with her white Keds. I noticed her left ankle was bandaged in a blue-and-white plastic brace. She seemed to ignore the pain and used both feet to scurry away.

I looked on after her and wondered who she was. I wondered why she was so dirty and why she left such an impression on me.

I wondered, then, if that was the woman my mother talked about. I wondered if this woman was Irma Smith.

I FED MY father dinner that night and went home. I drove in the Volvo, smoking out the window. I tried not to think of anything too deep on either side of feeling mournful or feeling frustration. It was always a battle, it seemed, though there was something about that floor that was different—about those patients and my father that seemed different. Something about the way he sat in that chair, banging it every now and then, and the way he now seemed to just spend the majority of his time staring straight into nothing.

Where was he going? And wherever it was—was he already there? I threw my purse on the counter in the laundry room, took my shoes off and was about to leave them on the mat before I remembered my mother's screaming the other day, and I put them back into the garage.

As I passed by the family room, I heard the television set to something in Italian. I didn't stop, but kept walking until my mother called out to me from the sofa. "Stefa? Did you see Irma?" She asked, turning down the volume of the TV.

I almost ignored her, but stopped.

"Isn't she so funny?" My mom continued, sitting up and facing me. "She is always so dirty. Did she talk to you?"

"Yeah, her breath smelled."

My mother scoffed and looked back at the television.

"She asked me if daddy was my father," I added. I didn't want any friends on that floor. I had already tried this once before with Adeline,

Evelyn and Cleda—even Pat and Buck. What was the point? My father was in a nursing home. I didn't want to care about anyone else.

"I work tomorrow. I'm going to bring her lotion and lipstick," my mother said as she lay back down.

I looked once more at her before turning to walk up the stairs and then stopped.

"Ma?"

"Yeah?"

"Wake me up tomorrow when you go—I'll come," I said and then went upstairs to my room and shut the door.

Chapter 24

Changes seemed to happen so fast that fall in 2003, but my father remained stuck in that corner beneath the picture frame that was now dented. While at college, I was beginning to find footing and family with Dan above me and Meagan beside me. She had gotten a new girlfriend who moved in with us—and though I was jealous, she had told me, "But if I didn't have her—I would hardly have you. You have Dan now—" she had said, as we sat together on our sofa weighing the pros and cons of having another body move into our basement apartment. I really couldn't argue though. Upstairs, Dan and I had our own separate sofas, though at times we shared one, and one ashtray between the two of us. But it seems there was always one for me and one for him—whether it was a sofa, or an ashtray, or a painting we each did on one of Dan's themed get-togethers.

"I was supposed to return this cable unit—because they're giving me all these channels for free! But yeah—I forgot to and now they're charging me," he said as he sat on his couch one day, slouching in front of his laptop, with a cigarette in one hand.

"Dan! Why do you always do this! This is how they get you," I said, annoyed. At times, I just wanted to shake him—but then I'd look at him again, stress flowing off his shoulders with the thoughts that mattered—"life goes on"—and then he'd be fine. Swallowing the mistake, he'd move on.

And that seemed to be my biggest test of all—swallowing always my own mistakes and trying to move on. My dad even used to say, "No es para tanto." In Spanish he'd tell me, tell my mom, tell Flavia—"No es para tanto" with his lips pursed and his eyebrows arching. "It's not a big deal," I should have told Dan—but I knew my father would never have said that—or my mother—or Flavia for that matter. "No es para tanto" only worked in the simplest of circumstances. Trying to think of a scenario now makes me think that perhaps it was just said as a joke after all. After all, if money or being taken advantage of were at stake—"No es para tanto" would never have been said. There would have been a lot of yelling and a confrontation. Maybe he always used to say it really, then, to joke with my mother. To push her buttons when she'd start getting angry about something and he'd want to tease her—from a little girl's perspective, I think that might be more of a likelihood. Especially when the little girl's parents seemed to fight often—maybe this "no es para tanto" actually worked as a Band-Aid more than anything else.

I never told Dan about that phrase—about the memories I have of it and the spaces in between where now I can only guess—or even ask my mother, of course. Dan and my father may have gotten along after all. Sure, they had their battles—but Dan represented a freedom that was so foreign to my family. Especially to a man trying to protect his family while the grip of his dementia began to tighten.

And never did it let up; it seemed to grow even tighter once that tray table over his geriatrics chair locked in place. His banging on the surface and the way he'd kick up his legs frightened me as I'd try to calm him, "Shhh, daddy. What's the matter? It's OK." And when it wouldn't work, I'd just sit back and watch him, trying to memorize his every movement.

I had been writing about what was happening now more than before. Before, I would write my feelings down in poetry or jotted down notes in scribbles. They would be my screams about missing Giuseppe in ways I didn't miss my father and vice versa. The feelings would flood the page and I would cut and know what I was experiencing was real and not imagined. But it seems that once my father reached the fourth floor nothing else mattered to me. All I could do was watch him, writing down the placement of objects and people and where and how things came to pass and it seemed that told more of a story and captured more my feelings than any words I could have invented.

And in those moments when my eyes were filming each twitch of his eyelids and hair follicle on his arm—she would always be there, the second I paused; she'd be again by my side. Ms. Irma Smith.

"Hi, Daddy. Are you hungry?" I said, as my mom helped serve lunch to all of the patients around me one weekend in September. She was so fast, so dependable, so personable with all of them. To Irma, she gave a glass of milk, then turned to me as I mixed up my dad's mushed up peas, chicken and whatever else they had served him. "Stefa, go get Irma some coffee."

I slowly got up from my chair and walked clumsily towards Irma after filling the cup of coffee. "Here, Irma."

"Thanks," she mumbled coarsely under her breath as she awkwardly grasped the cup in her hand. She began to pucker her mouth before the cup was even lifted from the table, bowing her head down to reach it. My smile appeared autonomously as I watched her.

Spoon-feeding my father was a bit difficult—I never knew how much to fill up the spoon before putting it into his mouth that either awaited food or was more or less kept closed. At times, I felt like I may have rushed feeding him, at times I felt perhaps I gave him too much at once just to be done with it. I still don't know if it was the chore of feeding him that got me most—or the idea that I was actually feeding him. Sadly, it may have indeed been both.

"Lloyd—here is your coffee. Do you want me to cut those pieces smaller for you?" My mom's voice came from behind me, to a man she had also grown attached to, Mr. Lloyd Weber. He was my father's neighbor in the corner and a sufferer of Parkinson's Disease. A former professor, in the final throes of the tremors that choked him as he ate, and yet he remained an avid listener.

"Thank you, Enida—I'm fine," Lloyd stammered as he moved his clenched fingers towards the peanut butter and jelly sandwich that he was given daily. His skin was white with wisps of faint, pale hairs along his arms and head. He had a button nose and eyes that watered and sparkled simultaneously. When he spoke, his voice often came out in gasps of air, or shaking, shallow tones and was often followed by his coughing.

I always tried to start conversation with him—but it never really went far. Not as far as my mother, who came home in the evenings at times, with news from Lloyd or stories she never finished—"Lloyd and I talked for an hour while Daddy was sleeping—" she'd say. "Lloyd told me to read this book," she proclaimed, holding a beat-up copy of *Man's Search for Meaning* up to me before going to her room with it.

Lloyd never ate much of his dinner, and what he did eat he'd mainly spit back up into a napkin that lay on his lap. His bib was promptly put on him by either Nicole, my mother or me, and always my mother would remind us, "Don't forget his lap—put one on his lap." When I first fed my father and saw Lloyd there by my side, I never understood why he came out to eat at all.

He had a feeding tube I watched a nurse use one evening as he lay on his bed, bent and jerking, trembling—like a small boy in a man's body, frightened by the sounds of his own suffering. It wasn't until later that I realized how much of himself he still had in him and how much of himself he had left to share with my mother—and the rest of us.

Irma didn't sit alone like my father and Lloyd—instead, she shared a round table with a few other women. The tall woman with a southern drawl had a habit of jiggling her teeth in her mouth when she wasn't talking about the fact that she was deaf. "Oh honey—I just woke up one mornin' and my hearin' was gone! Just like that!" She told me more than once. "Oh and you wouldn't believe my legs—oh! They hurtin' real bad and I just don't understand it!" She'd carry a small dry-erase board and prompt others to write on it at times so she could better understand the words she couldn't hear.

Across the table from her was another, smaller Ruth with brown, shoulder-length hair. She had a quiet and fragile face and she, like my father, was bound to a geriatrics chair. She never spoke and hardly ever moved without the help of a nurse's aide.

Irma would always look angrily at the quiet Ruth during mealtime, as her food would sit untouched. "Ruth, do you wanna die, Ruth? Why don't you eat? Do ya wanna die?" Irma would ask her, before turning her own eyes again towards her food.

MY MOM SAT with Irma after a while that evening, and pulled her wheelchair out to face her. Irma had finished eating, sitting with her dirty hands in her lap, or running them through her hair. "Irma! You are so dirty!" My mom exclaimed as she took a napkin from the box in the center of the table and dipped it in water.

I watched her quickly wipe the folds of Irma's face and hands, thoroughly cleaning away the debris of lunch and dinner that had buried itself on her skin. Afterwards, she said, "Irma, let's show Stefania the makeup I got for you," as she grasped a flowered makeup pouch that sat beside the tissue box.

"Yeah! Yeah! Put my lipstick on. Put my lipstick on!" Irma cried as my mother looked at me and laughed. While my mother went through the purse, pulling out lotion and massaging it into Irma's face, Irma asked, "Did you work today?"

"Yes, Irma. You know that," my mom said.

"How much they pay ya? Do they pay ya five bucks an hour?" I laughed under my breath as my mom looked at Irma with such love in her eyes.

Irma smiled as she waited for my mother to open the lipstick. And after a moment, contented and clean, Irma sat quietly with her painted lips, glancing up at my mother, who then came over to my father and me.

"Stefa, daddy lives now with Lloyd. I told them, I said Giovanni cannot stay with that other man. It smelled so bad—anyway, Lloyd likes to go to his room after dinner. Can you see if he wants to go now?" I looked quickly at Lloyd, who was staring out the window with food strewn about the edge of his plate and lap.

"Lloyd? Do you want me to take you back now?" I asked him nervously.

"Yes, please. Thank you," he said slowly, trembling as he turned his head to face mine. I removed his bib and cleaned off his lap as I wheeled him into his and my father's room.

"Do you want the television on?" I asked him.

"Yes—the channel is already set," he said as I made my way to the television, turning it on and then standing a moment, unsure of what to say or what to do next.

"Alright—goodnight, Lloyd. I'll see you tomorrow," I finally said. I was hesitant to leave him but also grateful to know that I could. It was difficult to know where to stand, what to say, but somehow my mother knew everything exactly—knew innately all the right things and all the right moments to do them.

As I made my way back down the hall and into the common room again, I saw my mother cleaning up my father's corner, his table and his shirt. Taking off his bib, she wiped his face clean and stood just a second and did nothing but watch him.

"Stefania? Go home. Go see what Nicole is doing—see if she ate. I'll come home in a little bit," my mom said as I stood beside her. I was feeling so unsettled there. And my mother could sense it I'm sure. I was beginning to understand how unnerving it could be when you're the only one who isn't.

"OK mom," I said, again thankful knowing I could leave, though I was beginning to also understand how unnerving leaving could be as well.

THE NEXT MORNING, I had woken up early, hoping to catch my mom before she left. I wanted to join her, since I would be leaving for school in the evening again with Dan.

My mother's face was sullen as that morning she drove. She seemed to be thinking, and I knew it was about her husband. She was thinking, and I knew it was about driving there—again. Her hair was flattened, and the crinkles at the corner of her mouth were drawn. Out of habit, she kept her glasses resting snugly on her head—so often she kept those glasses on her head, even Irma had started asking my mother almost daily, "Can you see better with your glasses on your head?"

"Ma, I want you to listen to this—here, put this CD in," I handed her a CD with no markings on the front, only now because I can't recall them. I can't remember the music I chose but it was some Italian sort from the sixties or the seventies—even the eighties or later. I had started to love doing things for her, to assuage her need for control and trick her into listening to me and trusting me.

"No, Stefa—come on!"

"Mom, just listen to it—"

"I don't feel like it, please!" She said, raising her voice.

But I ignored her as I pushed play and watched her as the car filled with the sounds of music playing gradually, growing louder—turning my mother's face more bright.

"You like it, Ma?" I asked as I smiled after her, seeing her hands start to keep rhythm on the wheel and her shoulders moving slightly to the sounds.

"I used to love this song, Stefa," she told me as I finally sat back and watched her come back to me. I listened to her sing aloud, watching her gain momentum and volume as she sang the chorus line, nearly screaming it.

I looked at her and followed her lead—just like I had and would continue still in the nursing home.

And in the midst of her singing, she turned to me slyly to serenade me. I watched her as she pushed the button for the sunroof to let in light.

I started moving my own head to match hers, and my whole body felt lighter, felt warm, felt free. It was like she was a bird, flying high now with the words pumping louder and the sun and the wind whipping through her lovely dark hair.

She thanked me with her eyes and grabbed my hand, holding it tightly within hers.

"DID YOU WORK today?" Irma asked me after my mother and I had arrived.

She was sitting slumped once again in her wheelchair. She had just spilled applesauce all over her lap. Her shirt lay like a slop trough, and no one had yet bothered to clean her.

"I worked at Wal-Mart." I lied. Really, I wouldn't have to work again until Thanksgiving break. But it was just easier to say yes.

"How much they pay ya?"

I turned to face her again, and take a pause from my father. "Eight dollars an hour."

"They pay ya five bucks an hour?"

"No, Irma. They pay me eight."

"I worked at Famous-Barr." Irma didn't look at me as she told me. Instead, she turned to comatose Ruth and held out her palm towards her, saying, "Ruth. Do you want to die? Why don't you eat?" I looked at Ruth who sat motionless, not listening—perhaps not hearing.

"Did you work today?" Irma asked me as she wheeled over to me.

"Yes, Irma. I worked at Wal-Mart."

"I worked at Famous-Barr for twenty-two years." As she told me, my mom walked over and said, "Watch, Stefa."

"Irma, I went to a lot of bars. Which famous bar did you work at?"

Then, as soon as she took in my mother's question, Irma dropped her head down and laughed. Her laugh sounded more like a cackle, a sweet cackle showing her brown teeth that hung next to nothing in her mouth. She put her dirty hand once again through her hair, this time leaving a mass of porridge atop her head. My mom laughed with her and then quickly ran over to get a towel and clean her up.

"How much does gas cost a gallon?" Irma asked my mom as her face stretched to and fro with my mother's hasty scrubbing. Then quickly, when my mom had finished, she resumed, "Put my lipstick on! Put my lipstick on!"

I shook my head in affection and looked out the window.

AND WHAT I saw must have been the rising road as I glanced down, letting the pressure of my foot against his urn relax. We were passing by a bend in the road where trees grow and bushes fatten, where the chance of an accident rises and each time a car comes down, I catch my breath in my throat. This is where at times my father ran—when he wasn't ascending from farther up the mountain, up near Il Girone where he once stood beside la Madonnina. But here, on this road, he would have been more cautious, since the cars were more numerous traveling up and down the mountain.

I wonder if I imagined him there in his white tank, inscribed perhaps with "Cozumel" or "Puerto Vallarta," with some sort of colorful outline of a coast or even a toucan. We'd pass by him, beeping I'm sure, banging on the windows and laughing. I would turn my head to face his, and look into his eyes and not turn them away as I had done. I'd keep them steady and sure and will him to keep going, and he, I'm sure, would do the same for me.

But he stopped looking at me back in the Alzheimer's Unit, right around the time his feet began to shuffle and his eyes lost control.

There was one thing that didn't change, really ever. And if I could return to that image in the car, staring into his eyes and he into mine as we passed by each other on the mountain, I'd include perhaps this one bit—him perhaps tripping or falling suddenly, and saying, "Naggia Cristo"—and the follow up, "Naggia la Madonn," both very bad to say, as I've learned in the cobbled streets in Pacentro. Both damning the Virgin and her son—but both so addictively enhancing to any rough situation or struggle.

So when the words left him, they did leave some residue—but of only these. The nurses in the Alzheimer's Unit grew fond of them. "Oh! John told me a new one last night—Va Fonc—" she started, a woman from the Philippines, telling me and my family one evening after he had been put to bed or as we awaited him being changed.

We would repeat the story to our friends back home, wondering how in the world he couldn't say "I love you" but could tell you to "fuck yourself" as clear as I imagine him once more running up the mountain.

So when my mother called me as I sat in the kitchen of my apartment at school, watching Dan struggle with the microwave, I didn't think it *too* out of the ordinary when she started, "Oh my god, Stefa. You will never believe what happened tonight!" And laughing, she continued, "Me and Nicole were sitting on either side of him after he finished eating and Nicole started asking me, 'how do you say do you want to leave now?' And so I told her—'Ce ne vogliamo andare,' and we both kept saying it over and over—she saying to me and me saying it back to fix the mistakes, you know? And then! Out of nowhere, daddy said, 'Ma vatten' a fongul!'"

"What!?" I exclaimed as Dan turned around with his hot meal steaming in his hands.

"Stefania, he said it so clearly! Me and Nicole were shocked!" she said, and then her voice returned to normal. "Then he just turned off again, and sat there, and didn't say anything or do anything else."

We both grew quiet, playing the scene over and over again in our heads, of him telling both of them off in annoyance in such a clear and familiar way. And giving them reason to hope for just a second that maybe . . .

"Stefania, Zio Mario is coming to visit dad," she continued, and I believe it was perhaps that same evening, though it could have been another night. But it was all the same, really—the message would have stayed the same.

His brother was finally making the journey back to see him, finally believing that he was sick. He would be coming with their youngest sister, Emma, who had visited him once before, back when he could still talk a bit more, walk a bit more and pretend still more.

"He is?" I asked, my whole demeanor changing, my eyes, I'm sure, growing dark as I began to fiddle with the sides of the round table.

"Well, good—about fucking time," I must have said. More angry than I could have thought I'd be.

Dan sat down beside me at the table as I stared at the telephone after hanging up. "What's the big deal?" he asked.

And I looked at him and I knew—I knew it was wrong to hold a grudge. I knew that in the end, it didn't matter and it wouldn't matter to any of us.

Instead of trying to explain my anger and frustration, I just watched him blow at the hot and scorching something he was eating. Finally, we found reason to laugh and did so wholeheartedly.

Chapter 25

I had forgotten my textbooks at Bethesda that night before they came to visit. I had left the books on the table beside my father in the corner of the common area. I didn't realize it until the day they arrived, after we had eaten dinner.

And so before I knew it, I was soon swirling into the scenes of earlier that day while I drove on that road that leads to Bethesda. I can still drive there in memory, passing the gas station on the left on Clarkson, that long, steep road past my psychologist's office, the library and finally another gas station at the corner of Clarkson and Manchester.

And I would have put in a piece of gum and chewed it hastily because of what happened once in the Alzheimer's Unit. My father cringed and his face contorted into such displeasure one day when I had happened to breathe onto him too strongly. At least that's what I thought—he had smelled my putrid breath from the stale cigarette I had smoked before coming, and it had made him recoil in disgust. Maybe it was something else though—a pain of some sort or a reaction set off by another set of cells dying. Maybe instead of cringing at my breath, it was really another sign that somewhere in his brain, another piece of him had disappeared. I spat out the gum in a trashcan near the elevator and walked past the fish tank.

IT WAS JUST hours ago—maybe three, perhaps more—that I had walked out of the same elevators and shunned the light from outside, turning my head downwards as I walked towards the common area.

I had driven haphazardly, lost in thought and forgetting at times to yield before turning, before switching lanes. My mind was elsewhere and my body wrenched with worry.

Zia Emma had visited a couple of years before, back when my mother first told them all he was sick. All that I retain from that visit is her standing in the kitchen, holding a handful of pills for her own illness she'd had for years, saying, "Look at all these pills. You think your father has a lot? Look at these . . . "

And my uncle never came. Not until he got word from others in the family that he was really sick, that he was in a nursing home, and that he was seemingly near the end. Thus it was my anger that kept me quiet upon first walking up to my mother and Nicole who, along with Irma, surrounded my father.

As I neared her, Irma looked up at me. "Is that your father?" she asked as usual, motioning towards our father with her palm out-stretched, though bent and arthritic.

"Yes, Irma," Nicole said, making eye contact with me.

"I was born New Year's Day. 1912," Irma continued.

"Wow! Irma, where does your niece live?" Nicole prodded.

"My niece Sandra Weber has power of attorney over me. She lives at the Ozarks. Is that your father?" She continued.

We laughed and I glanced at him, wondering what the day was going to be like in just a few minutes when the others would come.

"Did you work today?" Irma asked me, looking down at her lap, not really caring about the answer.

"Yeah, Irma. They paid me five bucks an hour," I said, grinning at my mother, who stood up and walked towards her.

"EEErma—I am from EEEtaly!" My mom said loudly as Irma looked up at her and laughed. Irma cackled and then gave way to small, high-pitched sounds making their way up from her belly and out her mouth. She looked ecstatic when she laughed—truly beautiful once more. Like the picture of the woman she kept on her dresser in her room, she would become again the younger Irma with the pearl necklace and red lips.

"I wonder what they're gonna say," said Nicole, her irritation and annoyance so fluid inside her, though she never really knew her uncle or her aunt.

"I don't know, Nic. But I can't wait," I said or may have thought without saying—I was simply stewing in my anger and spite for all the years they didn't believe us. Until now. I was salivating at the thought of my Zio Mario feeling remorse and guilt of such depth and weight that breathing may have even been difficult.

It was as though that dry and rough hand I felt across my cheek that day as a child never left me—the feeling I had when I heard him say, "She didn't cough once"—and the moment we locked eyes briefly before I coughed once more, again and again still more. And it was the same feeling I had when I imagined my mother crying into her open palms, covering her face that afternoon she hung up the phone after calling him and telling him the news about his brother.

I had placed my entire weight against the image of him and let it fall down to a level so deep within the hatred I carried for him. It was through the layers of time that I had forged such anger at my uncle that I had even written a story about him in a class once—it was a creative writing class my senior year in high school.

I had written a short piece about him, about a fictitious wife and fictitious son—and a man with early onset Alzheimer's disease. My uncle plays the man in the story who has just been diagnosed and is grappling with the illness, while his son shows no remorse and his wife only cooks and cries. In the story, my uncle, a repairman as in life, with gray and thick hair, hands so rough and coarse like sand and stone, kills himself one night as it rains outside his garage. He shoots himself as he sits at his desk beside broken-down refrigerators and torn-apart television sets. And for reasons I could only imagine, he couldn't fathom the idea of himself breaking apart, and decides that he is the type of man to end it before the real terror has yet to begin.

And I kept the story in my closet because Flavia told me I had the information all wrong, as she always seems to do even now—though I had told her again and again that it was just a piece of fiction. "Why are you still angry? Who cares, Stef? You need to let things go," she told me one day, after I had asked her to read the story. "Seriously, Stef. You think too much about it," she had said. And I let her words glide over my heavy shoulders for the most part, watching them fall down that same steep cliff where the image of my uncle lay.

I WAS GOING to be seeing him again for the first time since Nonna Concetta's funeral. I can't see him then in my memory; only now as I try to recreate that morning in the nursing home do his specifics start appearing. What I see is the hallway down where the elevators stood, and an outline of a nurse standing by her cart of pills and a nurse's aide or two walking past the first glimpse I have of my uncle. In a split second, I found myself finally in the moment I had waited for so long. I had been hungering for my father's family to acknowledge what he had been going through—what *we* had been going through—together. It was validation above pity that I sought.

So I tried not to miss a thing—not one step or blink. I memorized it all and later wrote it all down. It was like I had myself standing before a knife I held against my skin, forcing myself to remember everything, and in the process I seemed to have forgotten to feel it. Instead, I looked at the faces and the steps and imagined how we looked from their eyes—from his, my uncle's eyes, especially. I imbedded the way Zio Mario's eyes looked dark from down the hall and the way he seemed shrunken and the way he seemed too thin. In my childhood memories, he had always towered over me, frightened me. But as I stood there, touching my father's arm and seeing from my periphery, his moving hands and kicking feet—I noticed how small Zio Mario seemed to be.

He wears a white short-sleeved shirt now in my mind, and it's buttoned up for the most part, except right near his neck where a gold chain shows through. He walks with his arms to his side, and I see his top two or three teeth because his top lip is curling as he approaches the common room. I imagine his breathing becomes harried as he gains more of a view of the patients and his younger brother there in the corner.

He leads his timid sister, Emma, who stoops slightly as she walks dutifully behind him. Her short blond hair clashes with her brother's black and white sandy hair. Her eyes seem more drawn at the edges, but just like her brother, her eyes are dark and her lip almost curls.

I can still feel a bit of it all—feel the cold run through my body like jumping feet first into water bespeckled with ice, feel my breathing grow shallow and fast like it does when I near an accident and feel the rush of mortality sweep through me.

And they entered just so, seemingly transplanted out of the air and onto the fourth floor, like ghosts gradually materializing into skin and bone. Not until I went home later to write how it all finally happened did I add emotion to their steps, seeing instead their slithery approach as they entered into the common area, gliding past the tables with the women who sat scattered about like guards before my father. I imagined the woman in her flowered sunhat who sat tearing paper feel cold as they passed her and her tablemate with the frowning face must have surely felt startled the way my uncle and my aunt paused a second to look at her, considering for a moment if her frown was directed at them. But I would have to realize I had invented this momentary interaction as I sat cross-legged on my bed that night beside my lamplight.

But they did pass by her—I know that because I followed the same path each time I'd visit him. And so I transplanted my uncle and my aunt upon that same tiled route, and just as they pass her I turn the frowning woman's head with her sharp nose indignantly raised as they keep walking on, growing more timid still. And perhaps they picked up the pace the second the screaming woman bent back her head as she cried when my uncle stood directly opposite her. And perhaps that is when my aunt jumped and almost called out for her brother, who walked on by the screaming woman, who suddenly grew silent and began weeping. And was it then that the friendly woman who wore glasses and spoke of nothing else besides her dead daughter stood a minute longer than usual to let my uncle and aunt pass before making her way back to her bedroom? She would have shut her bedroom door the second Irma would have lifted her head to meet my uncle's face, which at that point would have glanced over at Lloyd, who was already watching him, steady as a switchblade.

But in my notes of that afternoon, Zio Mario's mouth was closed and his steady stare wavered as he came towards his brother. I made no mention of the others sitting there around us that afternoon. And Zia Emma, it seems, started crying back when she first saw us from the other side of the room.

Then it came—the reaction I had hoped for—from his brother, who was the first to break the silence. I had wanted him to feel floored, to feel the need to hold onto something sturdy else his legs would buckle beneath him. I wanted to see it in his eyes—the disbelief and finally the realization. I wanted him to feel guilty for having waited so long to believe us. I wanted his reaction to overcome him and for him to show even just an ounce of the weakness that his youngest brother showed us now daily without disguise.

"Giovann—o! Giovanni!" Zio Mario called out, and as I looked down at my father, I saw his eyes were closed. He often turned his eyes away or closed them entirely, evading interaction as though it were the sting to his ailment. I don't believe he controlled it—but the fact that his eyes happened to be closed the moment Zio Mario called out his name must have burned my uncle. It was all I needed—if nothing else were to happen, and he would have left, it would have been worth it.

Quite suddenly, I hear myself from the background of that memory. "Daddy! O! Giovanni! Daddy!" I said, shaking his poor shoulder, stroking his back, "Daddy?" The walls within me had begun to crumble. My shoulders were hunched, I'm sure of it, as I felt the mortar melt as Zio Mario began to weep.

And then, clearly, I remember Zia Emma looking at him, asking her brother if he recognized her. And I see her eyes were glistening and I wonder why she seemed so composed when I had thought for sure that she'd react much more severely.

But the way it did indeed happen seemed much more fitting, as it wasn't supposed to be my aunt to show me her sorrow and regret—it was supposed to be my uncle. And it was.

"Hey, Giovann—" he said as he grasped my father's shoulders tightly. I watched him as his own shoulders trembled with his heavy sobs that sounded like my own at times.

At this point in my notes of that afternoon, I had written down that I imagined I saw tears sliding down my father's cheeks as Zio Mario held him with his face against his shoulder. I heard Zio Mario whine out loud for a time, heard his sorrowful words that came out muffled against my father's tee shirt, and I imagined I saw my father looking towards the man he finally recognized as his older brother.

This whole scene only lasted a few minutes before we decided to move everyone to my father's bedroom. We were cramped standing there and the emotions were too thick and taking up too much space in that small corner.

Flavia pulled our father's chair behind her, as it was easier to maneuver that way. I held Nicole's hand as we followed Flavia and my uncle, who walked right beside my father's chair. Just as we approached my father's bedroom, I watched Zio Mario grab a hold of his brother's hand. And I saw my father grasp his brother's hand in return. Yet still he didn't look at him—but he held his brother's hand tightly. I could see that, even after they went inside the bedroom and Nicole and I were the only ones left inside the hall.

BUT DID I imagine it all? I'm sure it must have all been real—all of it playing out synergistically around me and before me. Even in his bedroom, I remember the light outdoors fading into blue and gray, lighting the contours of each one of us. And as I stood before the light that shone down on my father as he lay in bed, Zia Emma reached down her own hand to her brother's. But at this, he simply let her hand go. He let his arm fall onto the bed and began to twist and turn as Zio Mario stared out the window.

I could see Zio Mario's reflection from the doorway. He didn't say anything as he faced the window. He didn't make petty conversation or pretend to laugh or joke. He didn't try anymore to get my father's attention by calling out his name. He didn't need to. He was there to see him and say goodbye. He knew this, I'm sure of it—even if he didn't coming out of the elevator that afternoon. As he stared out the window, I wonder if he saw me watching him. I wonder, still more, if he knew his presence, the simple way he cleared his throat and the way he kept his arm against his back—I wonder, if he knew that his physical presence had reminded me that he was my father's brother. Perhaps I didn't realize it all right then and there in my father's bedroom that first day, but I knew it by the time he left. I could see us back in New Jersey—eating polenta around their table on a Sunday afternoon, he and my father sitting beside one another, yelling about a memory neither one could agree upon. After all of the simple signs I saw in him, the words he used to describe people and things, his strong emotions, the way he spoke with his hands, using the same gestures my father would—I saw them both in the ways that they were indelibly always different and in the ways that they would always be the same. He was the closest I could come to imagining what my father would have been like in ten years had this all been just a dream. I couldn't hate him. At least I couldn't any longer.

We only stayed in his room perhaps twenty minutes. It couldn't have been longer because when we left and said goodbye, there was still a bit of light left in the windows that surrounded him.

And so it was that after we had eaten dinner after coming home from their first visit to the nursing home, I went upstairs to my bedroom to find that I had indeed left my books at the table beside my father's chair in the common area.

I had been studying the day before, sharing a table with Lloyd. And though my intentions were good, I never really did manage to study much. Always, I brought some work with me to the nursing home, thinking, "If he just takes a nap or sits still for awhile, maybe I could do some reading," but then I'd start to daydream and lose focus and my eyes would fall again on him. And Lloyd, thankfully, was often there to bring me back.

"My mom said you lent her a book—*The Meaning of Man?* Was that it?" I had asked him once as I tried to study by my father.

"*Man's Search for Meaning,*" he said, slowly looking up at me. He had been sitting in silence since lunch and had since been breaking my heart.

"Why did you give it to her?" I asked him, trying hard to sound sincere but really knowing already all about the book. My mom had told me that she and Lloyd had formed quite a bond—that he had given her this book as a way to help her figure out how to endure it all.

"It helped me," he said. And I wondered if he meant it. Did he think back to these books that seemed to once in a while say something real and truly inspiring? Did he think of the lines he may have underlined once or twice as he sat for hours in the common area, with his bib still around his neck?

"Lloyd—thank you," I told him. I wanted to continue—and wanted to talk to him about his life and about how he found ways to continue helping others, especially my mom. I wanted to hear from him the stories he told her even though I could barely make out what he told me.

But all I had was a thank you and a smile and an offer to take him back to his room.

"You used to drive a Corvette, my mom told me—did you have one?" I asked, as I turned on the television and pulled his chair backwards until it was at a distance I thought comfortable.

"Oh yes, she told you that? I did . . . " he said, slowly smiling, his palms shaking so hard as his hands grasped the sides of his armrests.

I didn't know how to continue the conversation and keep it going. I tried hard to be like my mother—but I just didn't know what else to say. So again, I smiled as warmly as I could and left. I went and sat beside my father again and looked down into my book, and it surely didn't take too long before Irma came sliding up beside me, croaking,

"My birthday is New Year's Day."

"Is that your father?" she continued—"Sandra Weber has power of attorney over me," she said. And as I faced her, I wanted to do as Nicole had earlier that day. "EEERMA!" Nicole had said.

"Irma!! It's IRMA! Goddamnsonofabitch . . . " Irma had murmured. And Nicole and I had erupted in laughs. Our newest game had switched from simply applying lipstick on her and trying to make her laugh, to now making her angry enough to swear at us and then, after seconds, hearing her say "I love ya," as she'd fall back into her chair.

And then my mother's footsteps that Lloyd would say sounded like those of a state trooper had come barreling down the hall. "Eeerma," she had said, "Eeerma, you are so beautiful!" my mom had said as she looked at my father and studied his face, his clothes.

"Irma! It's Irma!" she cried, and then falling back into her chair, "Is that your father?"

"Stefania, they are coming tomorrow. Flavia is going to pick them up," my mom said as she straightened my father in his chair. He often ended up leaning either too much on the left or far too much on the right and then his bottom would slide down and he'd look so uncomfortable and so unsteady. My mom and I took out the pillow that we wedged beneath his arm and shoulder and straightened him up as Nicole turned to Irma, "Irma, did you go to the beauty shop today?"

"Yeah—yeah," she murmured as she sat up straighter, "I sat under the third dryer," she said as she began twiddling with her fingers before moving away, and rolling towards the table.

"Stef, I don't want them to come see dad. I mean I do—but—" Nicole started as she stood up. "I just think it doesn't matter anymore what they think. I hate them anyway."

"Nic," I told her as I sat down again and pushed my book back towards the window, "It's about damn time they're coming. They're assholes and I don't care either but god—I don't know," I started.

"What difference will it make?" Nicole asked. And really, what difference *did* it make—did I feel any different when they did eventually walk down that hallway? Did it all become more real? Did I finally feel vindicated?

I only felt more bonded to my family than ever—more centered in this place we had started to live within and breathe again within. And it was within that love we shared within those walls that I passed the window outside the elevators the day after, after the visit and the tears, with my head held up. I thought about my steps as I neared the common area—thought about how heavy they felt but also how sure and confident they were because I knew that whatever it was—whoever it was that I found at the end of the hall, I would be safe and I would be loved.

As I passed the nurses' cart, I saw him just as he normally looked. He sat, unmoving—just staring ahead of himself and kicking up his legs now and then and grabbing ahold of the tray on his chair.

I approached him and told him that we had gone home and mom had cooked us dinner. I told him I hoped he was alright and I told him I was sorry for what he had to go through that afternoon.

I stood a minute longer as I held the books I had gathered from the table underneath my arm. I contemplated leaving just like that, just after one "I love you" and having that be all. Instead, I leaned down to him, towards his cheek. I gave him a kiss. And he, my father, gave me a kiss right back.

I walked away, turning my head back every moment or so. I watched him over my shoulder as I passed by the nurses and the wall that slowly swallowed him up. He had kissed me goodbye. That I knew for certain.

Chapter 26

Just after the last turn, my uncle switched gears and accelerated. I saw the black and white sign that read "Benvenuti a Pacentro." We were getting closer to that picture in my mind with the gated village where the ghosts lived—inside that mausoleum where hopes lay buried. Outside those walls, loved ones anticipate their long-awaited embrace from the person whose picture stares back at them, smiling above the nameplate on the wall.

I watched the town as we approached from the backseat of my uncle's car. I wonder what expression I wore as I gradually accepted where we had finally arrived. I eased up pressure from my foot, relaxing it. I was now in the process of separation as we became entwined within the town and what thoughts I battled upon that journey, what fears I conquered, what sights I revisited I carried then as I looked towards the mausoleum to find the black wrought-iron gates ajar.

We didn't stop, but kept driving, passing beneath the shadows of the evergreens that lined the road. I watched the gravel dispersed along the dark street, and from either side of us, I noticed the bend of the branches and the clusters of wild flowers growing like moments of reprieve.

"Is it raining?" Irma asked as she wheeled herself over to me.

I glanced out the window behind my father's chair and squinted as the rays of sunlight came streaming in the common room. "No, Irma. It's sunny."

"Is that your father? Why doesn't he talk?" She asked as she parked her chair beside me. I attempted to answer her yet again, but just as I started to tell her he was sick, she switched focus.

"I went to the beauty shop today. I sat under the third dryer." She held her left hand in her right, playing with her ring that hung loosely around her ring finger.

"You look beautiful, Irma" I told her, seeing the difference clean hair made, though I knew that without fail, she'd put her soiled hand right atop her head at mealtime. "Irma, tell me about your family." I had already heard the stories over and over again but I wanted to remember every detail—I wanted to make sure I would remember.

"Rudy's my brother. He drowned himself in the river. Emily lived on a farm. I'm the youngest of eight children. Did you work today?"

"Yes, Irma," I said, disappointed she didn't go on to tell me about her parents, how strict they were, how beautiful Emily was. "Do you want me to put lipstick on you?" I asked her.

Irma quickly looked up at me and yelled, "Put my lipstick on! Put my lipstick on!"

After I garnished her in red, I rubbed lotion on her face and got her an ice cream. I sat beside her and told her about my job at Wal-Mart and played the game where I try to make her laugh. When I succeeded, everyone smiled—even the nurses. Everyone seemed to have opened up his or her heart to this woman, this slight questioner, Irma Smith.

Afterwards, I returned to my father. It was just days ago that he was visited by his brother and sister, and I had watched in anticipation as they reacted for the first time.

I had driven my aunt alone the second day they were here. Zia Emma wanted to come by herself, telling me in the car ride over, "I just wanted to come see my brother. That's why I didn't want Mario to come. I got two days—I was wantin' to spend all day with him. See if he knew me. I told Mario—wait by the elevator, let me see him first. And what did he do? He's walkin' right there in front of me."

"I really think it wouldn't have made a difference—he's the same with everyone," I told her. "It's not like he would have said anything to you." Then feeling guilty, "But at least you're going now with him. Zio Mario won't come 'til later with Mom. It's gonna be lunch time so you two can bond."

"That's great," she said. And then, after a while she turned to me as I drove, "God. You know your father—he was so funny growing up. He used to pull out his hair and pour it into his desk drawer while he studied. I says to him, 'Whaddya gonna do with all that hair?' 'Save it' he says, 'see how much hair I lose 'cause of school.' O—he was funny—joke after joke—everyone thought he was great."

I smiled at her in the car and couldn't think of enough ways to show her how important that little piece made—another layer I could recreate later when I needed to remember.

When we arrived, I went upstairs with her and took my father down to the dining room. I pulled his chair by the window and asked that his meal be given to him downstairs.

"I'll go home now—I'll come back in a couple hours," I told her, and she looked at me with what I could only assume was gratitude.

At home, my sisters and I stood in the kitchen beside the sink while Zio Mario sat alone at the kitchen table. He was talking to us about the years we were apart—about the ways in which he and my father eventually stopped talking. He talked about Nonna Concetta and how he and his wife took care of her at the very end of her life. I looked at him without really feeling bad for him when he told us about Nonna Concetta peeing on the floor and how she'd go into a rage at times—I wondered if he knew he was, in essence, describing his brother. I like to imagine there was an "I'm sorry" in there or a speech along the lines of that, but I can't honestly remember anything specific. Just stories from the past, really. That's pretty much all he had to tell us. But I couldn't hate him any longer. Still, I liked to dislike him. Brothers they were—just like my sisters and I. Except here was a lesson learned, one more lesson about familial love that stayed with me as I left shortly afterwards to pick up Zia Emma from the nursing home. I left knowing I loved my sisters more than I ever knew to love before.

I found them both upstairs in that corner beneath the dented picture frame. She seemed content, like she had formed a secret moment shared only between herself and him. And we were mostly quiet until we reached the car and she said without looking at me, "Your father cried when I fed him and he talked a little bit—said 'yeah' twice . . . Thank you."

And they left then, after the two days they were here. And again, I found myself where I often did, where I always did when at home. As my mother's footsteps came barreling down the hallway, I stood up and pushed the chair in. Flavia was going to be leaving for Italy after securing a rotation program at Boeing—she was to be working at the Italian office near Venice in Mogliano for several months. I wanted to be around her before she left—and I knew she was hesitant to leave, but my mother had assured her that it was the best decision—that it was time for her to move on, to secure a job and be successful. That, no doubt, would be his only wish.

As my mom approached she said, "Stefa go get the towels in daddy's bathroom. Get one wet with warm water and bring me his bag with his razor. I need to shave him."

I looked down at him as he looked forward, not really reacting to anything, but his legs moved just the same and he put his hands to his face like he often did. I went to his room and as I came back out my mother had already situated him differently, moving the pillow and moving his body so that he reclined comfortably.

I left her as she laid the warm towel over his face and he sat motionless. He must have loved that moment—he must have found a common ground where his varied thoughts and senses met and stopped with the stunning presence of warmth and comfort. As my mother lifted the towel from his face, I walked away, catching a quick and last impression of her as she smoothed cream over his face and studied him. I left them both and went home.

FLAVIA LEFT IN October 2003, just about a month after Zio Mario and Zia Emma left. She wouldn't return until the holiday. I believe it was Thanksgiving but it may have just been Christmas. Either way, it was when the weather was colder that time began to condense, and as I imagine now driving within Pacentro, driving towards the Piazza del Popolo and finally coming to a complete stop, I no longer panic. It's just a cool and calm sensation, like a warm towel spread over my own face as my reflection becomes his own. I remember the door opening and my foot leaving behind his urn for the last time as I stood up and onto the uneven surfaces of the cobblestones.

I can hear now the wheels of our luggage scraping against the ground as we walk together down the small hill towards our small street, Via Guardiola. I see the familiar sights I hadn't seen in nearly three years come to me in small bursts—the small statue of the Madonna against the wall of a home, the tunnel and the wall where Nicole had banged her head when she fell off her bike, and the final approach towards our wooden door.

Did I see Maria and Giuseppina sitting on their chairs outside Maria's cantina when we arrived? I don't think so—but I could be wrong. I could be imagining that that small section of Via Guardiola was quiet and all the sounds I did hear vanished as my mother and I came to a stop in front of our door.

And now I think back to that last night when Giuseppe had walked me home and given me a last memento to remember him by—a cassette of Smashing Pumpkins we'd listen to when we repeated the same versions of love that perhaps my parents had shared before. It was there, beneath our kitchen window, that we kissed amid our tears and he walked away and I closed the door. And it was there again that I found myself, only this time it was just as myself. It was just me, a daughter standing with her mother and the ashes of her father in a town that held the bones of their past.

It was just us inside our house, opening the window in the living room, changing the air and letting in light. And did I then go up the stairs and into the bedroom I shared with my sisters—opening those glass doors, letting up that finicky screen and finally, stepping out onto that balcony, feeling first the silken wind and then the thought that I was indeed right back there again?

Then I'm sure I would have heard my mother call me from downstairs, just as I had heard her call for me at the nursing home that day, his last Thanksgiving.

"Stefa! Don't drop the foccacia—Nicole, take the lasagna—bring it in the kitchen and ask them to give you plates," my mom ordered us as she held the small plate of turkey in her hands.

We didn't bring all the usuals—just our little versions of Thanksgiving—foccacia, lasagna, broccoli and turkey. My mom had brought enough to feed a few of her favorites at the nursing home, a few nurses and a few coworkers. We had also brought enough for one more—one special guest that I was sent to get.

"Irma! Happy Thanksgiving!! We are going to go eat turkey!" I said.

"How much does turkey cost a pound? Did you work today?" Irma asked, her head perked and her body restless.

"Daddy! Happy Thanksgiving!" I heard Nicole say as she wheeled him in front of me.

Nicole, my father, Irma and I all shared an elevator, and we talked and laughed our way to the dining room, where we found the table by the windows already set.

"Eeeerma!! Happy Thanksgiving!" my mother rang out as she took my father's chair, and I think I heard her say, "Happy Thanksgiving, Giovann'" as she wheeled him to the head of the table.

And we each took a seat; I fed my father as my mother fed Irma. And I faced Nicole, who laughed with me as a good-looking kitchen staff member who Nicole had a crush on—"Nursing home Ken"— came up to us and tried some lasagna. And we laughed still harder when Irma wouldn't stop asking between bites, "How much does turkey cost a pound?"

Still again, it was the same scene on his last Christmas—"How much does turkey cost a pound?"—as I filled our cups of soda in the dining area and my family sat at the table by the windows together, laughing and eating food we used to have back at home.

IN OUR HOME in Pacentro, I stood out on that balcony—whether it was before or after my sisters arrived, before or after we went to Zia Franca's house and saw her head hang over the railing and her quick smile before she buzzed us in—I went out onto my familiar balcony and stared out into those mountains and into that sky. By staring out into that sublimity, I was refilling my flat-lined senses again with the strength I needed should I find the will to scream if I needed to or cry if I couldn't. I had used up all of my energy in those few hours we spent driving to the town and finally ascending the mountain on which I now stood.

The air must have surely swept through my hair like it always did, and the vision of the Appennini and the distant Maiella surely must have stunned me initially. I had returned. I was back. And he, my father, was not.

I stood where he must have stood the last time he came with my mother. He wouldn't have been able to come out on his own—but I imagine her opening that stubborn screen for him and telling him to go out and stand a moment while she'd fix or adjust something inside. And he, barely moving yet quickly leaving, would have seen the same sights he knew so well. Perhaps he blinked back the intensity of it all, the sounds of life within the mountains, and the sights of living within such an embrace that comes from living with nothing but the hills and the sky and a slight terror from knowing how small you really are.

But even if my father felt small standing there—he was a part of it all—a part of that boulder painted in red, white and green in the mountain just across from where he would have stood—a part of those trees climbing upwards to the wooden cross mounted on top.

It was the last time he would stand and be so close to where he had come and where he would go, and yet he didn't know it. He would live forever and still be well, and yet none of us really understood it.

EVEN IRMA DIDN'T understand when I told her, "I'm gonna write about you one day."

"No. I have nothing to do with this world," she said as she turned away.

But her words wouldn't leave me. Maybe none of us have anything to do with this world. We live—having lived life, we die, taking our experiences with us.

But somehow, I still wanted to change this truth. I wanted to prove Irma wrong and prove the disease that stole my father wrong. Standing on that balcony in Pacentro, I wanted to bring back my father and uncover the moments like those when it was him standing on that balcony or at the side of a street, across from a statue of La Madonnina. But I knew I wouldn't be able to. Not then, anyway.

Because after the festivities, the mealtimes and the laughter, there we were at the nursing home again and again and again until shortly after New Year's Day, my father became ill. My daddy lay dying.

Chapter 27

"I was born New Year's Day, 1912," Irma loved to tell us. And finally, New Year's Day arrived. Flavia had just left again for Italy after our last Christmas spent together. Nicole was asleep New Year's Day morning because she had been with her friends. I had fallen asleep on the couch with my mother. We had fallen asleep to either *20/20* or a *Dateline* or some sort of news program long before the countdown began.

And at the sounds of neighborhood fireworks, my mother awoke suddenly and turned to me and asked accusingly, "Stefa—did you fart?" That was the height of our 2004 New Year's celebration.

But the next morning, I awoke early and drove towards the nursing home, hoping to find a card store on the way, to buy Irma a little gift.

I opened the door of a Hallmark store right between a Chuck E. Cheese and a liquor store. I had those goose bumps that fawned my skin whenever I came nearer to my father's residence. But at that moment, I was thinking of Irma and her smile and her awkward little movements. I was thinking of Irma sitting noisily beside herself in the common room, unknowingly celebrating her birthday.

"I'd like to buy a balloon please," I said to the woman behind the counter.

IRMA WAS SITTING in the middle of the common room, sulking in her chair. She seemed clean—cleaner than usual anyway.

"Irma! Do you know what today is?" I said to her as I turned her chair around to face me, holding out her "Happy Birthday" balloon.

"What's that? What's that?" she asked me, eyeing the balloon as it swirled in the air, captivating and red.

"It's New Year's Day. It's your birthday!" I tied the balloon to her chair, while she fussed around herself, trying to catch a better glimpse of her birthday surprise.

"It's my birthday. Is that mine? Lavagna? I was born on New Year's Day."

I laughed as I knelt down and gave her a kiss on her cheek. There was food on her face. I held back my disgust, and instead, wiped her clean and applied more lotion.

That's when I looked towards the corner to see him sitting, unmoving and quiet. His skin looked clammy, unwell. I sat beside him in a chair and took his weak hand in mine, pushing his fingers around my palm. I looked into his eyes and hoped he saw me. I didn't imagine he really had, but right then, it seemed enough that Irma had.

And moments later, I heard her strong, steadfast steps down the hallway. I heard her greet the nurses as she passed them. Then I heard her finally yell out, "EEErma!"

Irma raised her chin towards that familiar voice. "Irma! It's Irma!!" Then she saw my mother and smiled. "Anita. Did you work today?"

My mother laughed as she held out the two balloons she had bought for Irma. Smiling, we made eye contact, and then she turned quickly towards my father. He began to shake his tray, then raise his hand invariably towards his mouth.

There was nothing to be said, so we shifted back to the beautiful birthday girl. My mother tied her balloons on the opposite handlebar of Irma's wheelchair. Irma looked at us both as she told us once again, "I was born on New Year's Day. It's my birthday."

Then, when the excitement dwindled, she fell back into her chair.

EIGHT DAYS LATER Irma's balloons still danced atop her ceiling, sweeping over imperfections and cobwebs. It was 10:30 at night when the phone rang and I stood to answer. I had been lying on one couch, my mother upon the other, and we had both been nearing sleep amid the background sounds of the television when the phone began to ring.

"Hello?" I said, perhaps even in the same tone as my father had said it—when he received the phone call that would have changed his life forever.

"Hello, this is Cheryl from Bethesda. May I speak to Enida please?"

"She is sleeping. Can I take a message?" I said, a bit alarmed at the urgency in the woman's voice.

"John's disease has progressed—I think it's best that you all try to come down," she said as I began to panic. Without speaking, I went to my mother and held the phone out to her. My presence before her startled her awake as she took the phone, seeing my face contorted, my mouth open but silent.

AND THAT IS perhaps the moment my father's image melts again into my own as I stood on the balcony imagining him hours before his burial.

As I went back inside to the house, back through the window, I stood a moment in the silent bedroom that I shared with my sisters. I wanted them there right away—right as the breeze drew me once more to the mountains outside, to the white curtain flowing like a goodbye as I turned to go downstairs.

INSIDE THE CAR that night, my mother and I both cried, holding hands and wringing them. It was Flavia's twenty-fourth birthday that evening we received the phone call, and our worst fears were that he would leave us on that same day.

"Please—please not today," my mom cried as she grasped onto the wheel, staring into the windshield, out onto the road that led us to Bethesda. "Just a few more hours. Please, not now—not on her birthday . . ."

It was late that night when we finally arrived, parking quickly in that empty parking lot, save for a few cars owned by a handful of nurses and nurses' aides still on duty. I took in the sights as best I could, as though I would never again see the building from outside. It was like my mind began to memorize scenes that were especially important, and I can feel my head filling with details as I held on to my mom's arm and listened to our sturdy strides—the sounds of which I can remember even now. They were the sounds of our feared last steps into the building. I had to remember how to breathe and how to walk as we entered into the main doors, passing by the front desk and into the elevator.

I looked up at my mother's swollen eyes as we walked down the hall. She saw him first.

He was laid out on his chair; the tray table had been removed. It was as though he had a spotlight shining down on him. The light from the ceiling shone down on his unmoving frame in the front of the common room. He was pallid and his hands were cold. My mother cried anew as she reached down and kissed him. She went to speak to the nurses as I then approached him and held onto him—frantically looking all over his arms, his face, his hands—desperately trying to engrave him on my memory forever. His warmth I tried to weave into my dreams so that maybe I would never feel cold again, living alone without my father.

The pain I felt was so strange and awkward and strong. As I looked at my mother, who once again stood over her husband, I imagined she was doing all of what I was and more—fitfully trying to embed every last touch and sight within her. To never be alone, never without him.

And seamlessly within this memory, Nicole arrived with Linda. I don't remember why we came separately—perhaps she was sleeping over at Linda's house, or perhaps my mother had told her to stay behind and call for Linda. If anyone else would have been expected to join us in our last goodbye, it would surely be a Rallo—most assuredly, it would be Linda.

Nicole had walked on ahead of Linda, and I saw her eyes were like her mother's. She came to my father's side and looked towards me as I stood opposite her. "Steffy, is he dying?" She was hardly able to choke out the words. She sounded so small and frail that it was as though she were four years old, looking up to me, asking me a simple question. But as it was, I couldn't even begin to answer her—let alone even look at her without wanting to lie down beneath it all and pull the covers over my eyes and sleep. Nicole, though, wouldn't look away from me. She needed me to tell her something—anything—and so I nodded as I glide now, above the ceiling, rewatching this scene, watching her as she held on to him, softly calling out his name.

And then I pause and reflect upon that woman who walked in, her sure and quick steps coming towards us. I imagine she wore a clean and ironed white dress, but I could be wrong. She may as well have been in tatters, for what I can see is only the way she grabbed the chair from behind her and sat down. Her voice I can recall, jagged in its message and the hopelessness that it instilled in us—"He had signs of . . ." she started to say—"but I have no crystal ball," she finished.

Eventually she disintegrates and we are left again alone, surrounding him. I had gotten up to leave to call Flavia after my mother told me to. She had wanted to wait until it wasn't her birthday—wanted to wait just an hour or so more but she couldn't because we all feared he would leave us before then.

"Stef? Do you think I should come home?" Flavia asked me, her voice high and shaking.

"Yeah, Fla. Yeah—we all do. You should come as soon as you can," I said and then listened as she wept into the other line. I had never made her cry like that before—she hardly ever did anyway. To lighten the mood—even if just slightly, I started to tell her about the hospice nurse who still sat near the others around my father. "So there's this nurse who came . . . ugh, Fla. You shoulda heard her. She came and told us at least seven times that she didn't have a crystal ball," I quipped.

"What?" Flavia asked me. Suddenly she had stopped crying. "Why did she say that?"

"Well, we were asking her how much time he had—and I guess she just thought of that line on her way over and wanted to use it."

Flavia and I laughed together a little more until she told me she'd wait till the morning to buy her ticket.

After I hung up with Flavia, I sat down again beside Linda as we talked about him. We had started keeping vigil, it seemed, around him that night—in laughter and slight teases.

"I'll never forget the way he talked about his stocks—his stock dance," Linda said, looking over at my mother, who nearly snorted back—"oh my god, and that cushion. He would never stop telling me and Nick to save money and keep a cushion!"

Nicole's face brightened when the conversation shifted tone—we were freely discussing every quirk, every talent. "You know he could dance—he really danced well," my mom said.

"Well, he must have learned from all the traveling—all the places he went to, it's amazing," Linda said, her eyes beaming.

"Oh yeah—the traveling. Stefa you remember when he had an office in Mexico back when we lived in Erie? You remember Cesar? He used to work with daddy over there? Well, Nicole, you will never believe this. When I was in labor with you, Daddy was on the phone with Cesar in Mexico and when I was in pain—you know, in *labor*, he puts the phone up to me and says, 'Here—Cesar wants to say something to you'"—she started, and we all erupted. "I said to him—'Ma va fongulo!' I was so pissed!"

"I wish I could have met him when he was younger," Linda said.

"Oh you would have loved him—You know, Mama Concetta found marijuana once in his desk when he was in high school."

"What! Are you kidding me!?" I yelled, dumbfounded.

"Yes—are you crazy? You know, when we got married we had neighbors in Texas. We used to go there and he would go upstairs with them and come back down, his eyes red, and he was so weird. I told him he better stop and that I didn't want to go to those damn people's house anymore. I hated it!"

"I can't believe it! Then why'd you get so mad when I tried it!" I said, smiling.

"Stefa, don't start . . . " she said.

And as the stories dwindled down, the tone subsided and deepened as the time neared when we should leave. Nicole and I would go home together and wait for my mother's phone call if he should go in the night. We could come back in the morning, she told us. Linda would drive us home so we could sleep.

As we stood, Nicole and I took turns alone with our father. We each gave him a kiss on his damp skin that seemed drawn taut over his face. We touched his skin again and held his hand. Linda came by and stroked his cheek and then we left. We left without knowing if we'd see him again alive. We left without knowing what to think or expect of the night.

Nicole and I lay together side by side in our parents' bed. I waited for her to fall asleep so that I could go outside and sit awhile on my own. Nicole had wanted me to stay by her side the entire night; she didn't want to be alone for a second. And I couldn't blame her. I didn't want to be away from her either. But as I listened to her breathing become deeper and slower, I snuck out of the bed and down the stairs, taking cigarettes and a phone outside with me.

I was going to call Dan. I was going to tell him that he was finally dying. I was going to tell him that after the grief and sadness there was a bit of relief I felt growing.

I was going to tell him all, which I did, but only after I sat a few moments in silence, looking up at the night sky, at the stars, awake and staring to the moon, alive and blazing. I spoke to family members who were gone—who lived in the spaces between dreams and hope, nestled between the darkness and the light. I felt them all around me, my grandmothers and grandfathers, relatives I never knew and friends I had long ago. It was as if they were all there, meeting and congregating above us. I imagined that they were all there that night, keeping my mother company as she sat alone with him, keeping

Nicole warm in the bed I had left her in, keeping me safe and steady on the doorstep outside our home.

THE NEXT MORNING, my father was still alive beside my mother, though they weren't in the common room. They sat inside his room all night, my mother in a chair between her husband and Lloyd. Nicole and I arrived early that morning. We were tense as we entered his room, not knowing what to expect when we saw him.

He had changed since the night—he was no longer as pallid looking, as pale. He was lying still, however, and he was still not eating, nor drinking. He had pneumonia and it was causing infections and there was a fine line he was on between living and dying that no one seemed to really understand.

The hardest part of that illness was when mucus would overflow from his mouth, his nose. From somewhere inside him, he was drowning in his fluids, and it wasn't until one of us would start yelling for the nurses to come with their machine that would suction it all out, that his mouth would be clear again. These were my moments of a nightmare I dreamed over and over again and the moments that were the scariest. Those visions of him that he would never have wanted us to see.

Lloyd told my mother during the night that life is a mystery, not a problem to be solved. I couldn't think about anything else except how to solve the problem of whether or not I was going to say a eulogy at his funeral—and if that, what in the world was I going to say? How would I start? These questions were beating away inside my mind as we sat together in his room, watching him struggle to breathe.

When we went back home that afternoon, I took a shower, a long one, and tried to rid my boggled mind of the hours I spent dreading a speech I had yet to conceive of. I was thinking only of the end—as if I had been dropped to the bottom of the sea and was starting to swim back up, up towards the light I saw as it hung over me, blurry and yet promising. Was this all going to be ending? Was he going to be free now? Were we?

That night, Flavia arrived, and she went straight to the nursing home with my mother. Nicole and I stayed at home and waited for a phone call from the two of them. But again, the phone call never came, and again, we held our breaths before entering his bedroom the next morning. Six days later we heard the news that a grandmother of a neighbor friend of ours, the grandmother of Nicole's childhood friends, had passed away. It was she who ended up dying that January. We, instead, were told that "John's heart is as strong as an ox." And he soon got better; he soon ate again and drank again. He soon returned once more to that corner in the common area, feet away from where he lay just a week before.

Flavia stayed several days, just in time to watch him recover and return to his place beside the others.

"Did you work today?" Irma asked Flavia, one afternoon.

"Irma, I live in Italy. I work in Italy," Flavia told Irma, as we waited for the familiar response.

"In Illinois? You work in Illinois? What's your name?" Irma asked, though she had already done so moments ago.

"I'm Flavia."

"Flossy? Flossy, is that your father?" Irma asked, pointing her upturned palm with her bent fingers towards our father, who sat quietly across from her.

"Yes, Irma," Flavia said as Irma fell back into her chair.

We returned to our daily routines after Flavia left. Our father had gotten well, but no one was really rejoicing. It was the strangest feeling. And it lasted until that April, when we would all finally get what we had prayed for.

Chapter 28

The morning my father passed away, my breath smelled of bananas and coffee. I was not a fan of either, but Linda Rallo had come to the nursing home that morning. She had brought Nicole to my father's room to meet my mother and me—we had spent the night with him, me between my father, who was breathing shallow and sporadic, and me grasping his hand, grasping my mother's hand, hearing her tell him, "It's OK, Giovanni, you can go."

I believe it was the beginning of the week, perhaps a Tuesday, though it could have been a Wednesday just the same. I know this because the weekend before that day I had left my University to be with him. I was in my bedroom that Thursday evening, anxiously awaiting the morning when I would leave for Washington, D.C., with several friends to protest and march for the rights of women, for reproductive freedom, for gay rights and the like. It was a sponsored trip, organized by the Women's Center at the University of Missouri in Columbia.

I hadn't even told Flavia or my mother, though I did tell Nicole. I was just going to leave in the morning, leave and do something that they would never approve of or understand. Of course, Nicole would have. She was in seventh grade, the grade I was in when I first started slipping, when I first looked at my mother, who looked at me with more fear than understanding the day she picked me up from school to take me to my first psychologist. But Nicole was different. She was active in school, in living largely and laughing. Her clothes were stylish, her mind alert. She was beginning to care about the world and society, and her lust for speaking up for rights and the like was just starting to find a place in her own heart. Nicole was so jealous about my trip, asking me in jest, "Stef! Can I come? Why do you get to go and not me?" I was proud of her—she hadn't let herself become her enemy. She had, I realized, learned from my mistake.

Flavia remained a motherly influence, though she was without doubt my friend. It would be a year until our closeness was cemented, when I would study abroad in Bergamo, just an hour or so from where she lived in Mogliano.

It was Flavia who ended up calling me a few days before I was to leave. When I saw her name spring up on my cell phone, I nearly ignored it,

"Yeah?" I asked, as I lay on my side, staring into the purple and black tapestry I hung on the wall.

"Stef? What is this about you going to Washington? Are you nuts? You didn't even tell mom!?" She was worried, tense and angry, her trademark condition. Seven hours ahead of me in Italy, somewhere in her bedroom, she lay on her bed watching the sunrise behind the blinds in her bedroom. Somehow, she had gained the strength to find my actions once again capricious and erratic.

"Fla, can you stop? I just don't understand. I am twenty years old. When are you going to get that?" I started, gaining speed and anger, trying desperately to say something meaningful and convincing.

And then, in an instant, all the world paused for just a moment, even the waves themselves. "Daddy isn't doing well, Stef. They say this is it." I hadn't heard those words since January—when I had been the one to tell her. She had left a week or so after coming, and nothing had happened except we all realized we were, in a word, disappointed. Zio Mario ended up coming again with Zia Franca for one last visit. And then three more months would go by before my father would again lay dying. And if it weren't for Flavia calling me that night—I wouldn't have known in time before I left the next morning.

Flavia spoke with her voice a bit lower, a bit slower. "You need to call mom—you need to go home, Stef . . . I'm sorry," Her tone was one of calm acceptance. In a way, she was telling me *for* me since it was I who had been and continued to be too emotional, perhaps even too attached to his illness and our heartache. I would need the closure, need to see it to really believe it. I would need to see him leave us, kiss the wind goodbye and feel it.

I paused for a second, feeling more like minutes, tearing me like hours do. "Stefania. Stefania, just stop crying. Come on, I'm going to try to be there when I can," she told me soothingly. Again, she was carrying my burden, our burden. So far away from us, and she was holding me together and trying to ease my moment of guilt before it set in.

"But Fla, how do they know this is it? Remember last time?" I quickly imagined that past January when the nurses had told us all his time was running out. The scene had seemed illuminated in something more than the white light of the common area as we sat in a circle around him.

And when he did recover, when his fever broke and he was back to sitting dazed and agitated once again, I could sense the regret hanging heavy around us all. Flavia returned to Italy unsure of what to feel exactly, and we returned to the nursing home. And from time to time, we would mimic the nurse who regretted not having a crystal ball, and we'd joke to pass the time and laugh to lessen the strain of waiting. It seemed the misery of waiting became the prelude to the ending that would lead us somewhere else, somewhere warmer, somewhere familiar.

WHEN MY SISTERS arrived that afternoon in Pacentro, we all left the house together and said our goodbyes to Maria and Giuseppina—"Ma, come sei cresciuti!" They exclaimed at Nicole's sprouted height. Flavia and I were shorter than Nicole by a couple of inches, and somewhere in between stood our mother. We walked by the Bussis house where a door was open, and the sounds of yelling and loud conversations from within the house rushed past us. I don't believe my mother yelled to the women inside, because I imagine our walk was mostly silent, save for a few comments and exclamations, since neither Nicole nor I had returned to Pacentro for three years. We were making our way to Zio Marco's house, where Zia Franca was busying herself, preparing plates of prosciutto and cantaloupe, laying out fresh mozzarella balls and pasta; bread, she sliced while she'd yell to her daughter Flavia to go set up the table. When she'd think we were finally nearing, she would have yelled, "Sono gia arrivati,'" pleased we had arrived but hiding it in the hustle of preparations.

We entered the Piazza del Popolo after walking up the cemented incline from our street to the square. The flower shop was open and I could already smell the scent of the mausoleum's walls. Women, I'm sure, must have sat on the stoop outside the shop. We must have surely stopped for a few moments to say our hellos, accept condolences and finally tell them all, "Ci vediamo al cimitero," telling them we'd see them at the cemetery.

We would have kept walking, the four of us, though tired from the long journey. We would have passed the large church and I would have felt an air of comfort in knowing it was still there. The large fountain, the spigots of water cascading down from all around its sides would have left a trail of sound behind us besides our footsteps as we walked further onwards. We would have passed Franca's restaurant, and would she have been sitting there the moment we walked by? I can't say for sure—though the remnants of summers past, when my father would sit beside my mother at the white plastic tables remained unalterable. That would be the memory imposed upon his true past—the one that breathes the moments of his healthier days when he grew alongside the lifelines of the rocks and the walls of the town.

As we walked down Vico Diritto, we passed by homes with potted plants on the balconies, and voices coming through the open windows as the cats that roamed the corners swept by us. And just as we neared the steps leading to my uncle's house, a ghost reappeared wearing a blue shirt and jeans.

"Sono un fantasma," he had uttered that first time he walked me home—and a ghost he had become as he tore away from me suddenly the fall afterwards. I had learned to let go of the hope he had hinted at—I had, by the time I saw him three years afterwards, learned that the sort of hope I really sought was never the kind he could give me.

"Ciao, Giuseppe," my mother greeted him first. We stood around him in a semi-circle, and my voice seemed caught between my longing heart and my knowing mind.

I could see his eyes had gotten larger when he first saw me. Maybe he didn't even recognize me at first—I couldn't tell. But I wanted to turn around—anything but stand there next to him and say hello. Yet there we were, stopped just steps away from Zio Marco's house.

It was as though time had rewound and erased almost all of us, though I knew there did still remain at least a shadow of us somewhere. Though most of us had already washed away with the water in the spigot down my father's street. When I leaned in for the customary greeting, the two kisses, the embrace, his touch upon me still jolted me. I tried to act as cool as possible, telling him goodbye with a quick close-mouthed smile before turning briskly away. I couldn't hide from Nicole though, who laughed and said, "OK, Stef—calm down." And Flavia who added, "Oh my god, you look like you're gonna pass out."

My mother had already reached the door when I looked down and noticed, again, that plate of food.

Zia Franca still left plates of leftover pasta, it seemed, as we neared the bell and pressed it. And seconds later, we heard the door from upstairs creak open and her footsteps upon the balcony. Then we saw her hair rushing forward as she bent her head over the railing and called to us, "E! Benvenuti! Mo vengo!"

And just as we had years before, we pushed open the door and walked into her foyer, hugging, as we often did, and disappeared up the stairs.

When I reached the top of the stairs after hanging up the phone with Flavia, I threw open Dan's door and found him on his striped burgundy sofa, working on a paper that was due later that day. And then I fell into him and held him; we sat together like that, holding one another as I cried into his shoulder.

"He's dying," I told him. "It's for real this time," I sobbed.

"Do you want me to take you home now?" Dan asked.

"I'll have to call Nick and Linda—but I think we can wait 'til tonight. You can go to classes today—"

"Are you sure? I'll take you now—" Dan said, looking at me intensely, without hesitation.

"Yes, I'm sure," I said, as I lay on my back behind him, resting my tired eyes as he went back to typing.

DAN DROVE ME home later that evening after I called Nick and Linda to make sure I had enough time—I didn't want to waste the day, thinking I had plenty of time like the last time.

Before we left, Dan packed upstairs, while in my apartment I went from my closet to my drawers, trying to think about what to pack. Meagan and her girlfriend followed me around the apartment and stopped at my doorway as I stared at my black dress shoes, contemplating whether I should pack them. It was Meagan who finally nodded, as my hands trembled.

I chain-smoked that night in Dan's car. The traffic lights and the signs on the highways, the lit buildings and the lines in the lanes blurred and swirled together as I tried to maintain my bearings. This feeling, one of fear, of longing, of expectation—and even one of hope—swelled in me, growing like a blister. And if I would just be able to find a way to keep it still and keep myself from popping it—I'd have a chance to keep what was inside at bay.

We pulled up to the parking lot—the one that I parked at on New Year's Day. The liquor store and the Chuck E. Cheese were still lit as Dan and I got out. I asked him if I could change clothes while we drove because I knew the stench of my cigarettes would be much too overpowering in my father's bedroom. I changed in the backseat as Dan stood outside and had his last cigarette. Moments later, we drove up to the front door of Bethesda.

"Thank you, Dan," I told him as I hugged him goodbye. He clenched his teeth together like my father used to do before I shut the door and he drove away.

I went inside, and I don't see anything else as I focus on remembering going up in the elevator and stepping out as the doors opened on the fourth floor. My father wasn't in his corner; I guess that's how I knew to go straight to his bedroom. There, I found my mother already lying beside him on his bed. Lloyd was asleep in his bed, and the curtain was drawn between them. I went and lay beside my mother.

"Stefa—what the hell did you eat?"

"Why?" I asked.

"Oh my god—you smell like a Chinese. Did you eat Chinese food?"

"Yeah—yesterday for dinner," I said, annoyed that she could still smell it.

"Oh god—go brush your teeth. There's toothpaste and a new toothbrush in the bathroom. I'm gonna gag," she said before making a slight retching sound.

I think I brushed my teeth and my tongue about three times before I finally settled in beside them. I hadn't gotten rid of the "smell," as my mother said, but I think she finally came to terms with it.

We took turns, my mother and I, lying beside him. For a while, I lay between the two of them and grasped my father's hand, staring at his silhouette and leaning against him, pretending he was leaning against me.

Neither one of us slept much—though my father didn't move. He kept his eyes shut the entire night. He had been sleeping for several days, off and on oxygen. That night I don't recall if the oxygen mask was on his face. I see him as clearly as I used to in my memory of that final night. I lay between my mother and my father, and it was as though it was how it was meant to be and always remain. I fell asleep at one point in the night holding my father's hand and when I awoke, I was smiling.

Towards the early morning, just before the sun had risen, my mother whispered in my ear, "Stefania, I bet Irma is awake. Did you ever see her when she is in bed? She's so cute—go see her, go see."

I agreed and left the bedroom, figuring it was better to give myself space from them. I walked down the hall and looked into an open doorway that my mother had said would belong to Irma.

And there she was. As I walked up to her bedside, she opened just one eye and then finally the other.

"Did you work today?" she asked me, in the same way she always did.

"No, Irma. I came to see my dad," I said as tears fell down my cheeks.

"Is it morning?" She asked again.

"Yes—good morning, Irma. It's morning,"

ONCE THE SUN had fully ascended, I was able to finally study him as he lay there on his white sheets. All his muscles seemed to hang like flab. I couldn't understand how his skin had gotten so thin and so fragile over the past year. And his legs had mainly withered away with scattered scabs dotting them plainly. He used to have strong, thick arms and he'd show off those muscles to me in his muscle tees whenever he jogged or stood beneath the sun on the beaches of Mexico. I never did see him lift weights—he seemed to awaken with muscle; it seemed to grow from within him.

My father had been on morphine for several days, and nothing but his eyebrows moved every so often. The only sounds he'd make came when he snored.

It was bright outside when Linda brought Nicole over to my father's room. My mother and I had long since been standing, sitting, hovering around corners in his bedroom.

"OK, I got bananas and I got coffee," Linda said as she handed each of us both.

"Hi Stef!" Nicole said as we hugged tightly. "I wish you would have called last night—I would have come too," Nicole said.

"I'm sorry, Nicky. Dan just took me straight over—" I said, feeling guilty.

"It's OK, Stef," she said, knowing that if she didn't, I'd dwell on it the entire morning.

Somehow, we drank all our coffees and had eaten our bananas. The cups and banana peels we had thrown away spilled over the edges of the small wastebasket beneath the desk that stood at the foot of his bed. A hospice nurse had come in at one point as we stood around my mother, who kept adjusting his oxygen, wondering why his fingers were turning blue.

"I'm not going into the biological processes anymore. Just take this time to be with him," he said, as my mother looked at him and realized what she had to do.

She took away the tubes from his nose, lifting his head gently as she took them away. And then she shut the machine off and wheeled it back. Nicole and I stood together at his side, my mother at the foot of the bed.

WE SAID GOODBYE to him that morning. Tremendous and unexplainable, the disease had long since left us hollow, but our final goodbye to him was saturated with all he was and all he would forever be.

The gates of the cemetery were ajar as we drove up and parked beside the entrance. My mother held onto his urn, which was made of polished wood, with his name engraved in gold. My sisters and I met up in a line behind her. We each held on to one another as we walked through the entryway made of white stone and entered into a space of open air. There were already people standing alongside the pathway to the Cappella di San Carlo where my father would be laid to rest. There were already women clad in black dresses, young people, friends of ours, standing in small groups on the sidelines, and others whom I didn't recognize congregating near the entryway to the Cappella.

Farther down the path, we followed our mother, past the benches lining the edge of the lane, laden with gravel and small pebbles. Pinecones littered the ground, fallen from the trees that shrouded the empty spaces.

We walked as one down the small path that passed the fountain where later we would stop to gather water for his flowers. We passed the small wall made of darkened stones cemented together in rough design that bordered the path on one side, where on the other, trees and small private mausoleums lined the edges of the cemetery.

It was on that pathway that he'd motion for me to follow him down to where his relatives were buried years before. It was on that same pathway that he'd lead me into the darkened corridor with the lonely nameplate, "Giovanni Silvestri."

I walked heavily on towards the stairs that led up to the second floor of the Cappella di San Carlo. I put my entire weight against my feet and heard the crushing and crinkling of the pinecones beneath me.

My sisters and I walked slowly up the stairs and through another set of open gates where a flock of women stood waiting for us. They had never seen an urn before; my father's was the first of the town. Many of them didn't understand it, some didn't agree with it—but they meant nothing to us really, those that only came for the spectacle. Really all that mattered in those last moments was us and the ones we loved. It was always like that, even at the nursing home.

AFTER OUR LAST goodbye, I sat beside myself in the hallway, crying into my hands as I sat cross-legged on the floor. And at one point, I slowly lifted my eyes from beneath my hair and saw her coming from a room down the hall on her wheelchair. I could tell how small Irma's hands were against her frame as she bent her neck low to look at us. My sister and Linda stood near the doorway of my father's former bedroom, and my mother was nowhere to be seen. Irma started to open her mouth; I nearly heard her voice. But before anything, a nurse came and wheeled her away, back into the common room.

Later, my mother told us how she had walked into the common area to say goodbye to Irma before we left.

"Irma, I love you. I will miss you," my mother said as she reached down and kissed Irma on the cheek.

"Did your husband die?" Irma looked into my mother's eyes and, my mother noted, sadness seemed to echo.

"Yes, Irma. He's dead."

"Now you're a widow like me," she said, as she fell back into her chair.

IRMA DIED NEARLY a month to the day after my father. She had passed away shortly after asking for a hotdog from my mother, who fed her in the common area for the very last time.

Irma, I'm sure, was on that journey with us and watched us as we walked out of La Cappella later that afternoon. The crowds had dissipated and the sounds were softer. The air was warm and tinged with the sweetness of flowers, of lilies, of roses.

All that was left was the dust and stones on the pathway of the cemetery, the scenes across the white marble face that bore his name. It was in the breeze atop the mountain that our journey seemed to finally come to an end. And in the times when I think back now, summoning up the scents and sounds of the days when all I had was fear and longing, I realize how so much has come and gone. Spiders crawl across his picture; the gold letters of his name become entwined in webs. At times, the rain splatters against his smile, falling in small beads, leaving rivulets on the surface. The flowers in the vase mounted beside his name sway silently with the wind, and petals fall slowly to the ground. It is like water over sand; like time. In essence, a memory.

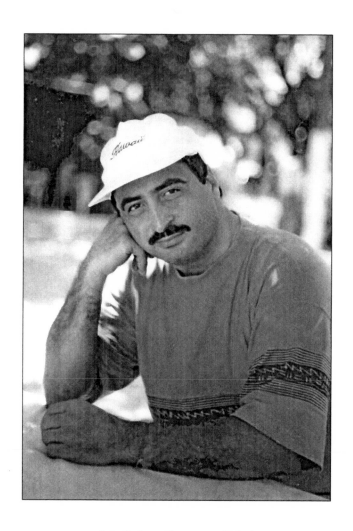

My father, Giovanni (John)

CPSIA information can be obtained at www.ICGtesting.com
Printed in the USA
BVOW041226120213

313046BV00001B/14/P